WOMEN'S ISSUES

MATERNAL MORTALITY

TRENDS, IMPACT AND REDUCTION EFFORTS

WOMEN'S ISSUES

Additional books and e-books in this series can be found on Nova's website under the Series tab.

WOMEN'S ISSUES

MATERNAL MORTALITY

TRENDS, IMPACT AND REDUCTION EFFORTS

MATHIAS T. GREGERSEN
EDITOR

snova
New York

Additional color graphics may be available in the e-book version of this book.

Library of Congress Cataloging-in-Publication Data

ISBN: 978-1-53618-161-6

Published by Nova Science Publishers, Inc. † New York

CONTENTS

PREFACE

Every year in the United States, hundreds of women die of complications related to pregnancy and childbirth. According to CDC data, racial/ethnic disparities exist with regard to these deaths. For example, non-Hispanic black women were more than three times as likely to die as non-Hispanic white women, and non-Hispanic American Indian/Alaska Native women were more than two times as likely to die as non-Hispanic white women. This book describes trends in pregnancy-related deaths in the United States, including trends in causes and timing of these deaths, and the efforts focused on reducing pregnancy-related deaths.

Chapter 1 - GAO's analysis of the Centers for Disease Control and Prevention's (CDC) Pregnancy Mortality Surveillance System data shows that from 2007 through 2016, over 6,700 women died of causes related to or aggravated by their pregnancy—either while pregnant or within 1 year of the end of pregnancy. While CDC data show an overall increase in the pregnancy-related mortality ratio in the United States during this time frame, the annual ratio fluctuated. Cardiovascular conditions, infection, and hemorrhage were the leading causes of pregnancy- related deaths, and comprised about 50 percent of all pregnancy-related deaths from 2007 through 2016. In addition, CDC data show that the leading causes of pregnancy-related deaths differed by racial ethnic groups.

Chapter 2 - This is an edited, reformatted and augmented version of Hearing before the Subcommittee on Health, of the Committee on Energy and Commerce, House of Representatives, One Hundred Fifteenth Congress, Second Session, Serial No. 115–169, dated September 27, 2018.

Chapter 3 - This is an edited, reformatted and augmented version of U.S. Department of Health and Human Services; Centers for Disease Control and Prevention; National Center for Health Statistics, Publication No. 2020–1428; Series 3, Number 44, dated January 2020.

In: Maternal Mortality
Editor: Mathias T. Gregersen
ISBN: 978-1-53618-161-6

Chapter 1

MATERNAL MORTALITY: TRENDS IN PREGNANCY-RELATED DEATHS AND FEDERAL EFFORTS TO REDUCE THEM*

United States Government Accountability Office

ABBREVIATIONS

AIM	Alliance for Innovation on Maternal Health
CDC	Centers for Disease Control and Prevention
HHS	Department of Health and Human Services
HRSA	Health Resources and Services Administration
MCH	Maternal and Child Health
MMRC	Maternal Mortality Review Committees
MMRIA	Maternal Mortality Review Information Application
NIH	National Institutes of Health

* This is an edited, reformatted and augmented version of United States Government Accountability Office, Congressional Requesters, Maternal Mortality: Trends in Pregnancy-Related Deaths and Federal Efforts to Reduce Them, Publication No. GAO-20-248, dated March 2020.

NVSS	National Vital Statistics System
PMSS	Pregnancy Mortality Surveillance System
PQC	Perinatal Quality Collaborative

WHAT GAO FOUND

GAO's analysis of the Centers for Disease Control and Prevention's (CDC) Pregnancy Mortality Surveillance System data shows that from 2007 through 2016, over 6,700 women died of causes related to or aggravated by their pregnancy—either while pregnant or within 1 year of the end of pregnancy. While CDC data show an overall increase in the pregnancy-related mortality ratio in the United States during this time frame, the annual ratio fluctuated. Cardiovascular conditions, infection, and hemorrhage were the leading causes of pregnancy- related deaths, and comprised about 50 percent of all pregnancy-related deaths from 2007 through 2016. In addition, CDC data show that the leading causes of pregnancy-related deaths differed by racial ethnic groups (See figures).

WHY GAO DID THIS STUDY

Every year in the United States, hundreds of women die of complications related to pregnancy and childbirth.

According to CDC data, racial/ethnic disparities exist with regard to these deaths. For example, non-Hispanic black women were more than three times as likely to die as non-Hispanic white women, and non-Hispanic American Indian/Alaska Native women were more than two times as likely to die as non-Hispanic white women.

GAO was asked to review issues related to maternal mortality in the United States. In this chapter, GAO describes, among other things, (1) trends in pregnancy-related deaths in the United States, including trends in causes and timing of these deaths, and (2) HHS funding efforts focused on reducing pregnancy-related deaths.

GAO reviewed documentation about HHS's surveillance efforts related to pregnancy-related deaths; and analyzed CDC data on leading causes of pregnancy-related deaths from 2007 through 2016 (the most recent 10-year period available at the time of GAO's review). GAO also reviewed documentation and interviewed HHS and state public health officials in five selected states about HHS's funding efforts aimed at reducing pregnancy- related deaths, including select efforts used in these states.

GAO selected these states primarily based on their geographic diversity and their implementation of select efforts to address maternal mortality.

GAO provided a draft of this chapter to HHS. HHS provided technical comments, which GAO incorporated as appropriate.

Pregnancy-related death, as defined in statute, is the death of a woman while pregnant or within 1 year of the end of a pregnancy— regardless of the outcome, duration or site of the pregnancy—from any cause related to or aggravated by the pregnancy or its management, but not from accidental or incidental causes. 42 U.S.C. § 247b-12(e)(3).

White and black women were non-Hispanic. Hispanic women might be of any race.

The Department of Health and Human Services has 13 ongoing efforts aimed at reducing pregnancy-related deaths. The following are key examples of these:

- Supporting Maternal Mortality Review Committees Cooperative Agreements. According to CDC officials, in September 2019, CDC awarded 5-year cooperative agreements to 24 recipients covering 25 states with amounts ranging from $150,000 to over $550,000 in the first year, totaling about $8.4 million. Under these agreements, CDC is providing funding to state agencies and organizations that coordinate and manage Maternal Mortality Review Committees. The committees are responsible for comprehensively reviewing deaths to identify prevention opportunities.

- Maternal and Child Health (MCH) Services Block Grant Program. The Health Resources and Services Administration provides funding through this program to 59 states and jurisdictions to improve maternal and child health. In fiscal year 2017, total expenditures for services for pregnant women from all sources—federal funds, as well as state, local, program income, and other funds—was about $300 million. According to agency officials, many recipients reported using their block grant funding to help support or complement other federal initiatives, such as their review committee, quality collaborative, and use of maternal safety bundles.

According to officials GAO interviewed in five selected states, they use these efforts and others collectively to address pregnancy-related deaths. For example, according to officials in one state, they implemented an obstetric hemorrhage maternal safety bundle in 2018 based on the state's Maternal Mortality Review Committee finding that hemorrhage was a leading cause of pregnancy-related deaths in the state. According to officials, the state's Maternal Mortality Review Committee was funded primarily through the MCH Services Block Grant.

All five states also mentioned beginning or continuing to address racial/ethnic or other health disparities with block grant funding, through their Maternal Mortality Review Committees, or other efforts. For example, officials in one state said they use block grant funding to support their Black Infant Health Program, which helps address maternal morbidity and mortality of black mothers in the late maternal period. Additionally, two of the HHS funding efforts awarded in fiscal year 2019 have outcomes related to decreasing racial and ethnic disparities in maternal mortality: the Alliance for Innovation on Maternal Health Community Care Initiative and the State Maternal Health Innovation Program.

March 12, 2020
Congressional Requesters

Every year in the United States, approximately 700 women die of complications related to pregnancy and childbirth, while thousands of others experience life-threatening complications.[1] In 2014, for example, more than 50,000 women experienced a life-threatening pregnancy complication, such as heart failure or cardiac arrest during surgery or a procedure. While the maternal mortality ratio decreased globally by about 3 percent from 2000 through 2015, the ratio in the United States has increased by about 3 percent for this time period.[2]

Within the Department of Health and Human Services (HHS), the Centers for Disease Control and Prevention (CDC) is the federal agency responsible for surveillance—the continuous, systematic collection and analysis of health-related data—of all deaths in the United States, including pregnancy related-deaths. CDC data show that racial/ethnic and age disparities exist in the rates of pregnancy-related deaths.[3] For example, from 2007 through 2016, non-Hispanic black women were more than three times as likely to die than non-Hispanic white women, while non-Hispanic American Indian/Alaska Native women were more than two times as likely to die than non-Hispanic white women (See Figure 1).

Similarly, rates of pregnancy-related deaths for women 35 years old and older are higher than the rates for women under 35 years old (See Figure 2).

---

[1] M. C. Lu, "Reducing Maternal Mortality in the United States." *JAMA*. vol. 320, no. 20 (2018), 1237-1238.

[2] For purposes of this chapter, we use the term "maternal mortality" broadly to mean the death of a woman during pregnancy, at delivery, or soon thereafter. The maternal mortality ratio is the number of maternal deaths—those occurring during pregnancy or within 42 days of pregnancy—per 100,000 live births, as defined by the Word Health Organization. "Global, regional, and national levels of maternal mortality, 1990–2015: a systematic analysis for the Global Burden of Disease Study 2015." *Lancet*, vol. 388 (2016) 1775-1812.

[3] A pregnancy-related death, as defined in statute, is the death of a woman while pregnant or within 1 year of the end of a pregnancy—regardless of the outcome, duration or site of the pregnancy—from any cause related to or aggravated by the pregnancy or its management, but not from accidental or incidental causes. 42 U.S.C. § 247b-12(e)(3).

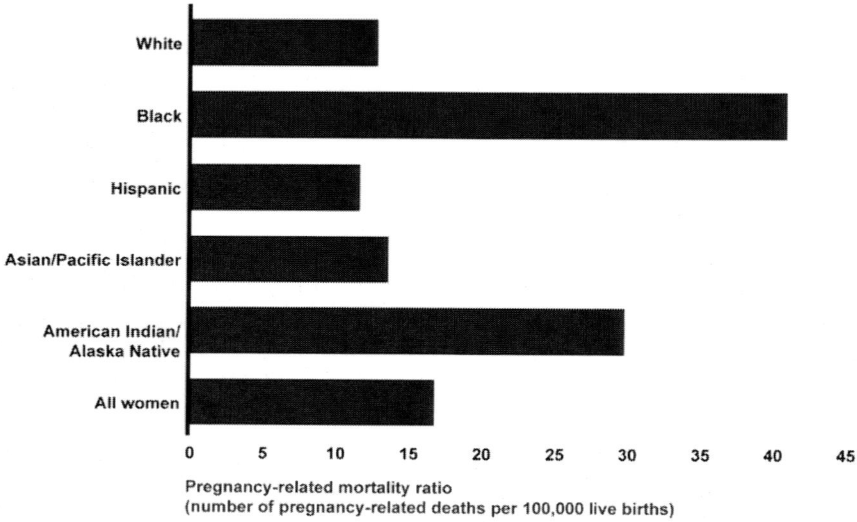

Source: Centers for Disease Control and prevention Morbidity and Mortality Weekly Report, September 2019. | GAO-20-248.

Note: White, black, American Indian/Alaska Native and Asian/Pacific Islander women were non-Hispanic. Hispanic women might be of any race.

Figure 1. Pregnancy-Related Deaths per 100,000 Live Births by Racial/Ethnic Group, 2007-2016.

According to a Health Resources and Services Administration (HRSA) report, access to consistent, high quality, and reliable data that identify both the characteristics of women who die due to pregnancy complications and the specific circumstances that lead to these deaths is essential to inform critical action steps and for developing prevention strategies.[4] Such data can inform, for example, state and local efforts funded by HHS to reduce these deaths.

You asked us to review issues related to maternal mortality in the United States. This chapter describes

1. HHS's surveillance efforts related to maternal mortality;

---

[4] Department of Health and Human Services, Health Resource and Services Administration, *HRSA Maternal Mortality Summit: Promising Global Practices to Improve Maternal Health Outcomes Technical Report* (February 15, 2019). HRSA is the primary federal agency within HHS for improving health care to people who are geographically isolated, economically or medically vulnerable.

2. trends in pregnancy-related deaths in the United States, including trends in the causes and timing of these deaths; and
3. HHS funding efforts focused on reducing pregnancy-related deaths.

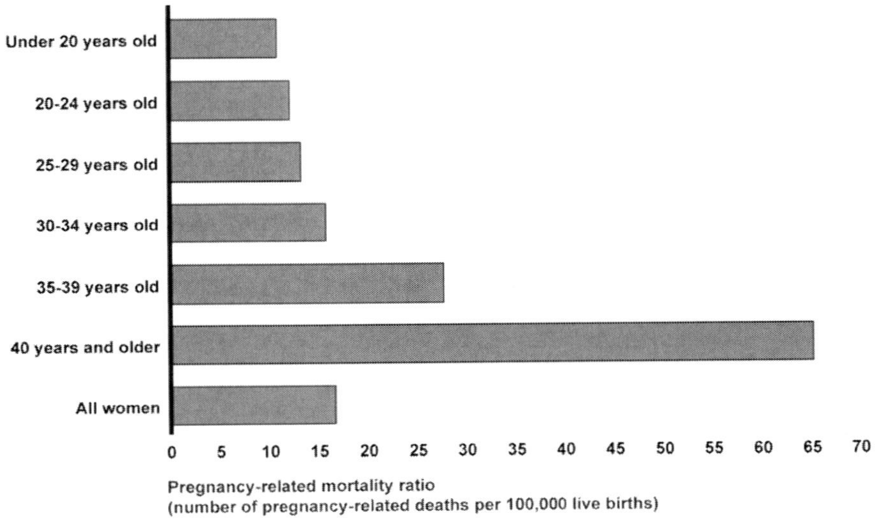

Source: Centers for Disease Control and prevention Morbidity and Mortality Weekly Report, September 2019. | GAO-20-248.

Figure 2. Pregnancy-Related Deaths per 100,000 Live Births by Age Group, 2007- 2016.

To describe HHS surveillance efforts, conducted by CDC, related to maternal mortality in the United States, we reviewed agency documentation, such as reports on maternal mortality. We identified three such efforts—the National Vital Statistics System (NVSS), the Pregnancy Mortality Surveillance System (PMSS) and the Maternal Mortality Review Information Application (MMRIA). We also interviewed CDC and selected state officials (see state selection criteria below).

To describe the trends in pregnancy-related deaths in the United States, we analyzed PMSS data, including any age or racial/ethnic differences, for these deaths from 2007 through 2016—the most recent 10-year period available at the time of our review. We also analyzed PMSS data on the timing of pregnancy-related deaths in the United States—whether the death occurred during pregnancy or within 1 year of the end of the pregnancy—for the period of 2011 through 2016. According to agency officials, data on this variable were not collected by CDC until 2011. We assessed the reliability of the PMSS data by (1) comparing PMSS data provided to GAO with published reports, (2) reviewing existing documentation on the data and the data collection processes that produced them, and (3) interviewing agency officials knowledgeable about the data. We determined that the PMSS data were sufficiently reliable for our purposes.

To describe HHS funding efforts focused on reducing pregnancy-related deaths, we reviewed agency documentation, such as agency notices of funding opportunities and award announcements, and interviewed officials at CDC, the Centers for Medicare & Medicaid Services, HRSA, the Indian Health Service, the National Institutes of Health (NIH), and the Substance Abuse and Mental Health Services Administration about their efforts to reduce maternal mortality. HHS officials identified these agencies as having efforts that may focus on reducing maternal mortality. For our review, we identified ongoing funding efforts with a stated outcome, goal or focus on reducing pregnancy-related deaths.

In addition, we interviewed state public health and vital records officials from five selected states—California, Georgia, Illinois, Maryland, and Texas—about their efforts to reduce maternal mortality. We selected these states because of their geographic diversity and because these states have

- a Maternal Mortality Review Committee (MMRC), which are multidisciplinary committees whose goals are to systematically and comprehensively review clinical and non-clinical information about pregnancy-related deaths to develop recommended strategies for preventing future deaths.
- a Perinatal Quality Collaborative (PQC), a network of multidisciplinary teams that work to improve measurable outcomes for maternal and infant health, and disseminate best practices.

- at least one of the maternal safety bundles implemented—sets of evidence-based practices that when implemented collectively and reliably in the delivery setting may improve patient outcomes and reduce maternal mortality and severe maternal morbidity—that were developed as part of the HRSA-supported Alliance on Innovation in Maternal Health (AIM) initiative.[5]

BACKGROUND

Death Registration Process

We conducted this performance audit from October 2018 through March 2020 in accordance with generally accepted government auditing standards. Those standards require that we plan and perform the audit to obtain sufficient, appropriate evidence to provide a reasonable basis for our findings and conclusions based on our audit objectives. We believe that the evidence obtained provides a reasonable basis for our findings and conclusions based on our audit objectives.

In the United States, deaths from all causes are recorded and tracked through a multi-step registration process, which may vary by state, according to CDC officials. According to CDC officials, when an individual dies, a death certificate is filed with the state. Funeral directors are responsible for providing demographic information about the deceased individual, while physicians, coroners, and medical examiners are responsible for providing information on cause of death. The local registrar of vital statistics is responsible for verifying the information, and then transferring copies of the death certificate to the city or county health department in some jurisdictions, and to the state registrar. The state vital registration office is responsible for verifying the information, maintaining official copies, and creating an electronic record. According to CDC

[5] Severe maternal morbidity includes unexpected outcomes of labor and delivery that result in significant short or long-term consequences to a woman's health.

officials we interviewed, state vital records offices submit their death certificate information to CDC electronically.

In 2003, CDC revised the standard death certificate to include a checkbox to indicate whether a woman was pregnant at the time of her death or up to 1 year after delivery or end of pregnancy (See Figure 3).

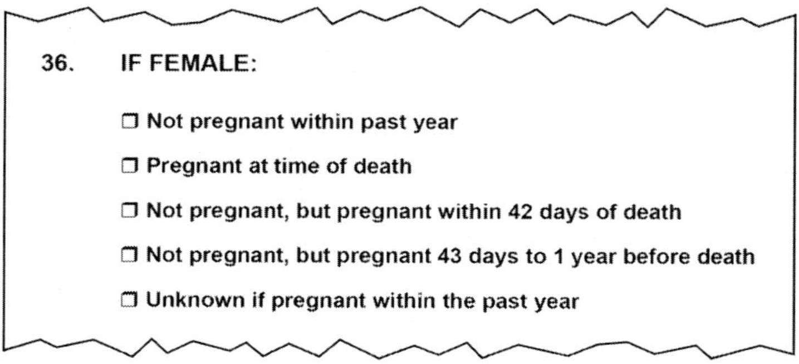
36. IF FEMALE:

❒ Not pregnant within past year

❒ Pregnant at time of death

❒ Not pregnant, but pregnant within 42 days of death

❒ Not pregnant, but pregnant 43 days to 1 year before death

❒ Unknown if pregnant within the past year

Source: United States Standard Death Certificate (2003 revision). | GAO-20-248.

Figure 3. Pregnancy Checkbox in U.S. Death Certificate.

CDC Has Two National Surveillance Systems Related to Maternal Mortality and Has Created a Resource to Facilitate State Efforts

The checkbox is part of the medical portion of the death certificate that is completed by a physician, coroner, or medical examiner. According to CDC officials, there has been staggered adoption of the revised death certificate by states, and not every state death certificate included the pregnancy checkbox until 2019.

CDC collects maternal mortality data using two national surveillance systems, NVSS and PMSS. In addition, CDC has developed a data application that state or local MMRCs can use to centrally collect information abstracted from various sources about each death.

NVSS

Federal law directs CDC's National Center for Health Statistics to collect statistics on maternal mortality.[6] According to CDC officials, the National Center for Health Statistics receives copies of electronic records for deaths from all states and jurisdictions, such as the District of Columbia. It uses this death certificate information to assign ICD-10 codes based on the cause of death.[7] According to CDC officials, the National Center for Health Statistics uses these coded records to compile national vital statistics files in NVSS, which is the source of official statistics on mortality in the United States, including maternal deaths.[8] NVSS data are used to identify national trends and make international comparisons.

CDC published national maternal mortality rates for deaths that occurred in 2007 based on data collected in NVSS in its report on all deaths in the United States.[9] CDC also made these data publicly available in microdata files that can be downloaded through website applications and, according to officials, in response to specific requests when additional details, such as geography, are sought.[10] However due to staggered

---

[6] See 42 U.S.C. § 242k(b)(1)(A).

[7] According to CDC officials, staff review and assign an ICD-10 code manually to these deaths because they are rare in contrast to most other deaths, which are coded using an automated algorithm. Starting in 1999, CDC began coding causes of death using the 10th edition of the International Classification of Diseases (ICD-10). ICD-10 includes a specific category (O codes) for pregnancy, childbirth, or puerperium-related causes of deaths. The puerperium period typically refers to the time after pregnancy when a woman's reproductive organs return to a non-pregnancy state. According to CDC officials, for a death to be assigned an O code, the death certificate must have indicated that the woman died during pregnancy, within 42 days of pregnancy, between 43 days to 1 year after pregnancy or included a cause of death that indicates one of these conditions. Within the O code category, there are codes for specific categories of causes of death, such as a code for postpartum hemorrhage.

[8] NVSS uses the term "maternal death," as defined by the World Health Organization, to mean the death of a woman while pregnant or within 42 days of pregnancy, irrespective of the duration and site of the pregnancy, from any cause related to or aggravated by the pregnancy or its management, but not from accidental or incidental causes. The term does not include "late maternal death," which occurs more than 42 days but less than 1 year after pregnancy.

[9] The maternal mortality rate is the number of maternal deaths—deaths during pregnancy or within 42 days of pregnancy—per 100,000 live births, as defined by with the World Health Organization definition.

[10] Through CDC's website, the public can access vital records data, including data on maternal mortality, using an application called CDC WONDER. According to CDC officials, through

implementation of the 2003 revised death certificate by the states and reliability concerns about the use of the pregnancy checkbox, CDC officials said that as of September 2019, they have not published NVSS statistics on maternal mortality in the agency's annual mortality reports since the report on deaths that occurred in 2007. For example, as specified in the technical notes of a June 2019 CDC report on national vital statistics for deaths in 2017, CDC noted evidence of an increase in false reporting of maternal deaths as a result of incorrect completion of the pregnancy checkbox on death certificates. According to CDC officials, the individual who completed the pregnancy checkbox may have incorrectly noted that a woman was pregnant or had been pregnant within 1 year of her death, and as a result, the death would have been recorded as a maternal death or late maternal death. However, prior to the addition of the pregnancy checkbox, there was a general concern that the United States was not identifying all of the maternal deaths and thus did not have a full picture of maternal mortality.[11]

According to CDC officials, the agency has recently taken steps to improve NVSS data on maternal mortality. For example, in 2018, CDC developed training for individuals who complete the cause of death portion of a death certificate, and in 2019 was developing guidance on completing the pregnancy checkbox. The agency also participated in a quality assurance pilot from January 2016 through March 2017 with four states, Georgia, Louisiana, Michigan, and Ohio, to test processes that may improve state-level data on maternal mortality. The results of the pilot were made available in articles in 2019, and CDC officials said the agency is currently disseminating the findings from the pilot to other states.[12]

HHS's Office of Women's Health's website, the public can access vital records data, including data on maternal mortality, using an application called the Health Information Gateway.

[11] For example, CDC officials noted some death certificates contain only general cause of death descriptions and do not contain enough information to determine whether the death was related to the woman's pregnancy.

[12] A.E.C. Daymude, A. Catalano, D. Goodman. "Checking the pregnancy checkbox: Evaluation of a four-state quality assurance pilot." *Birth.* (2019) 1-8 and Catalano, A., N.L. Davis, E.E. Petersen, et al. *Pregnant? Validity of the Pregnancy Checkbox on Death Certificates in Four States, and Characteristics Associated with Pregnancy Checkbox Errors.* (forthcoming).

According to agency officials, one of the findings from the pilot was that a greater proportion of deaths where the pregnancy checkbox on the death certificate was marked incorrectly were for women aged 45 and older. As a result, CDC officials said they plan to use additional criteria when classifying deaths for these women. Specifically, they will only code the death as a maternal death or late maternal death if the cause of death is explicitly reported on the death certificate as due to pregnancy or an obstetric cause.

PMSS

CDC officials stated that the changes they made improved the accuracy of data on maternal mortality, and they will implement the new reporting criteria for 2018 data.[13] On January 30, 2020, CDC published maternal mortality statistics in a National Vital Statistics Report.[14] For data on maternal mortality accessible through CDC's website, CDC officials said they will direct users of these data to its limitations that are noted in the annual report. Officials said they will also publish guidance on the limitations of the maternal mortality statistics, and they will continue to monitor the accuracy of the data. Taking these steps to improve the NVSS data on maternal mortality and noting their limitations should help provide federal, state, and local organizations with accurate data. For example, CDC notes on its CDC WONDER website that state, local, and county health departments rely on this source of publicly accessible data to review their community's population health trends, evaluate their program's

---

[13] In addition, CDC officials said the agency plans to release additional data files using the new reporting criteria for years 2015 through 2018 and provide those files in response to individual data requests for these years.

[14] Department of Health and Human Services, Centers for Disease Control and Prevention, *Maternal Mortality in the United States: Changes in Coding, Publication, and Data Release, 2018*, National Vital Statistics Reports vol. 69, no. 2 (Maryland: January 2020). CDC also published two related publications in January 2020. HHS, CDC, *Evaluation of the Pregnancy Status Checkbox on the Identification of Maternal Deaths*, National Vital Statistics Reports vol. 69, no. 1 (Maryland: January 2020) and HHS, CDC, *The Impact of the Pregnancy Checkbox and Misclassification on Maternal Mortality Trends in the United States, 1999-2017*, Vital and Health Statistics series 3, no. 44 (January 2020).

performance for planning purposes, and compare their community with other locations.[15]

In 1986, CDC initiated a second national surveillance system for maternal mortality, PMSS. Unlike NVSS, PMSS is exclusively focused on pregnancy-related deaths. According to CDC, the system was developed because more clinical classification of the causes of these deaths was needed in order to fill data gaps and help clinicians and public health professionals to better understand circumstances surrounding pregnancy-related deaths, including the causes and appropriate actions to prevent them. This collection effort included expanding the scope of deaths under surveillance to those up to 1 year after the end of pregnancy, which is beyond the international standard of up to 42 days after the end of a pregnancy.

To collect the additional data, CDC officials annually send requests to vital records offices for all 50 states and other applicable jurisdictions to provide the following: death certificates, linked live birth or fetal death certificates, and any other supporting information for 1) deaths with an ICD-10 Chapter O code for the previous year, and 2) all deaths from any cause (including injury or trauma) among women who were pregnant or were within 1 year of pregnancy as identified by matching the death certificate to a birth or fetal death certificate or by a pregnancy checkbox on the death certificate. According to CDC officials and related literature, linking information on death certificates to information on infant birth or fetal death certificates can help confirm that the pregnancy checkbox on the death certificate was completed accurately. In addition to confirming validity of a pregnancy-related death as indicated by the checkbox, linking information on death certificates to infant birth or fetal death certificates can identify pregnancy-related deaths where the checkbox did not indicate a pregnancy but should have (false negatives). CDC officials said that PMSS data are considered the most reliable source of national data on pregnancy-related deaths because (1) PMSS links death certificates with

[15] Information on maternal mortality is available on CDC's Wide-ranging ONline Data for Epidemiologic Research (CDC WONDER), which is a public resource—an application that makes many health-related data sets available to CDC staff, public health departments, researchers, and others. WONDER-508.PDF. Accessed on November 20, 2019.

birth or fetal death certificates and additional information when available (e.g., hospital records), and (2) these files are reviewed by medically trained epidemiologists to determine if the cause and time of death are related to the pregnancy.

CDC publishes national data from PMSS on the leading causes of pregnancy-related deaths and pregnancy-related mortality ratios using this system. However, the data are not published annually—such as is generally the case with NVSS data on deaths—and only national level data are made publicly available from PMSS in annual updates on the website and periodically in reports.[16] According to agency officials, states and jurisdictions voluntarily provide the records in response to CDC's request that specifies that PMSS analyses will only be published at the national and regional level, and those records are subject to confidentiality protections.[17] Additionally, according to CDC officials, because of the time involved in collecting documentation from states, the most recent data available from PMSS as of September 2019 were for deaths in 2016.

MMRIA

To improve the timeliness of PMSS data, CDC is taking steps to gain access directly to the records that states have been submitting to the agency. Specifically, CDC entered into a contract, effective August 2019, for a pilot project with the National Association for Public Health Statistics and Information Systems to become an approved user of the State and Territorial Exchange of Vital Events system.[18] According to the National Association for Public Health Statistics and Information Systems, this vital events system provides timely access to state vital records, including records on deaths, to federal and state data partners for use in authorized

---

[16] As noted earlier, CDC resumed publication of NVSS data on maternal mortality in January 2020.

[17] See 42 U.S.C. § 242m(d).

[18] The National Association for Public Health Statistics and Information Systems is an organization representing 57 state and other jurisdiction vital records offices that developed and operates the vital events system, a private electronic portal through which vital records information is shared among data partners, on behalf of state vital records offices.

public health and administrative programs, like those at CDC. According to the contract, over the next 5 years, select CDC staff will receive training on the use of the system and will coordinate phased access to state and jurisdiction vital records.[19] At the conclusion of the contract, authorized CDC staff are expected to have access to electronic vital records data from up to 51 states and jurisdictions. CDC officials said this should allow them to link birth and death certificate information and no longer rely on states and jurisdictions to conduct vital records linkages for PMSS.[20] According to CDC officials, being able to access the vital events system will allow them to confirm and report pregnancy-related deaths with improved timeliness.

In 2017, CDC released MMRIA, in which MMRCs—multidisciplinary committees at the state and other jurisdictional level that review pregnancy-related deaths—can collect and review data from various sources (e.g., medical records, social service records, autopsy reports, and vital records) to determine preventability, and identify factors that contributed to these deaths as well as prevention strategies to address these factors.[21] As of June 2019, CDC officials said that 25 states and one other jurisdiction were using this system.

While MMRCs provide the information collected in MMRIA, federally published reports only include aggregate information from select states collected through the application. For example, in May 2019, CDC published a study using information from 13 states.[22] In the study, state MMRCs identified an average of three to four contributing factors per pregnancy-related death based on information collected through MMRIA, such as:

---

[19] According to CDC, National Association for Public Health Statistics and Information Systems activities will occur as funding allows.

[20] Before this agreement, CDC's Division of Reproductive Health requested that states link the certificates and then submit the linked documents to CDC. According to CDC officials, some jurisdictions are timelier in providing information than others.

[21] The Maternal Mortality Review Data System was the precursor to MMRIA. Published reports on the results of MMRC reviews have included data from both systems.

[22] E.E. Petersen, N.L. Davis, D. Goodman, et al. "*Vital Signs:* Pregnancy-Related Deaths, United States, 2011–2015, and Strategies for Prevention, 13 States, 2013–2017." *Morbidity and Mortality Weekly Report (MMWR),* vol.68, no 18 (2019) 423–429.

- community factors (e.g., unstable housing and limited access to transportation);
- health facility factors (e.g., limited experience with obstetric emergencies and lack of appropriate personnel or services);
- patient factors (e.g., lack of knowledge of warning signs and nonadherence to medical regimens);
- provider factors (e.g., missed or delayed diagnosis); and
- system-level factors (e.g., inadequate access to care and poor case coordination).

Similar to PMSS data, the most current aggregated data that CDC publishes from the MMRIA can be for deaths that occurred 2 or more years prior to the date of the report. As noted in the May 2019 article, the most recent information from states contributing to the article varied with some state data on these deaths being as recent as 2017 while the most recent data from other states was from 2014. According to CDC officials, in August 2019, CDC awarded 24 cooperative agreements covering 25 states, and under these agreements, the committees will use the system to record review results within 2 years of a death.

DATA SHOW AN OVERALL INCREASE IN THE PREGNANCY-RELATED MORTALITY RATIO, WITH SPECIFIC CAUSES VARYING BY RACE/ETHNICITY, AGE, AND OTHER FACTORS

Cardiovascular Conditions, Infection, and Hemorrhage Were the Leading Causes of Pregnancy-Related Deaths, though Causes Differed Among Racial/Ethnic and Age Groups

Our analysis of CDC's PMSS data shows that from 2007 through 2016, over 6,700 women died of causes related to or aggravated by their pregnancy—either while pregnant or within 1 year of the end of pregnancy.[23] Our analysis also shows that while there was an overall increase in the pregnancy-related mortality ratio during this time frame, the annual mortality ratio in the United States fluctuated.[24] As previously noted, CDC data also show that racial and age disparities exist in the rates of pregnancy-related deaths. For example, from 2007 through 2016, non-Hispanic black women were more than three times as likely to die than non-Hispanic white women, while non-Hispanic American Indian/Alaska Native women were more than two times as likely to die than non-Hispanic white women. Similarly, rates of pregnancy-related deaths for women 35 years old and older are higher than the rates for women under 30 years old. During this time period, the specific causes of death varied by race/ethnicity and age. Further, CDC data show that most of the deaths occurred within 42 days of delivery or the end of pregnancy.

CDC's PMSS data show that among all pregnancy-related deaths, the cause of death varied. In general, what CDC classifies as "other cardiovascular conditions" was the most common cause of pregnancy-related deaths, followed by infection, hemorrhage, and cardiomyopathy.[25] (See Figure 4) These four leading causes comprised about 50 percent of all pregnancy-related deaths from 2007 through 2016. See appendix I for more information on leading causes of pregnancy-related deaths.

CDC data shows that the leading causes of pregnancy-related deaths differed by racial/ethnic groups. Specifically, for non-Hispanic white and black women, the leading cause was other cardiovascular conditions from 2007 through 2016; for non-Hispanic American Indian/Alaska Native and Asian/Pacific Islander women, it was hemorrhage; for Hispanic women, it was infection, as indicated by Figure 5. CDC has reported that multiple

---

[23] We based this information on PMSS data, which we found to be sufficiently reliable for reporting pregnancy-related death information at the national level.

[24] The pregnancy-related mortality ratio is the number of pregnancy-related deaths per 100,000 live births.

[25] "Other cardiovascular conditions" includes conditions that are not reported separately as cardiomyopathy—when the normal muscle in the heart thicken, stiffen, thin out, or fill with substances the body produces that do not belong in the heart muscle, or cerebrovascular accidents—also known as stroke. PMSS categorizes causes of pregnancy-related deaths into 11 categories. See Appendix I for more information about these categories.

factors contribute to pregnancy-related mortality and to racial/ethnic disparities, including community, health facility, patient/family, provider, and system factors.[26]

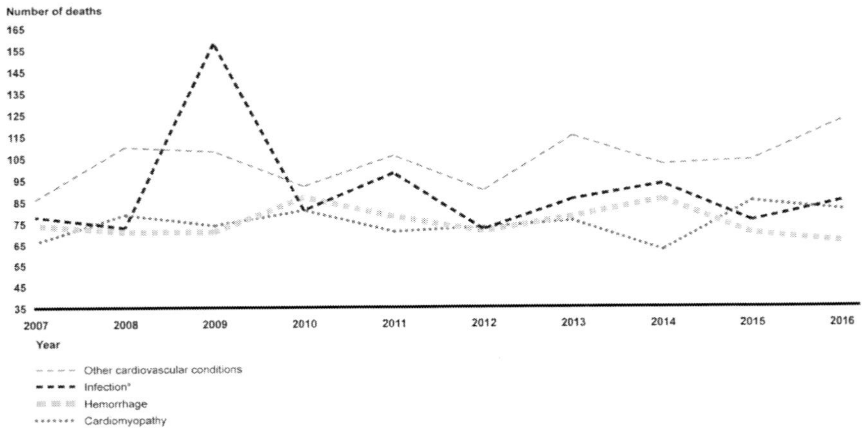

Source: GAO analysis of Centers for Control and prevention Pregnancy Mortality Surveillance System data. GAO-20-248.

Notes: "Other cardiovascular conditions" includes conditions that are not reported separately as cardiomyopathy—when the normal muscle in the heart thicken, stiffen, thin out, or fill with substances the body produces that do not belong in the heart muscle, or cerebrovascular accidents—also known as stroke.

In multiple CDC publications of Pregnancy Mortality Surveillance System data, "other non-cardiovascular medical conditions" is a leading cause of pregnancy-related deaths. GAO did not include this category in the figure because the category is composed of more than 10 diverse conditions, including cancer, autoimmune disease, and gastrointestinal disorders, among others, that each represent less than 3 percent of all pregnancy-related deaths for the 10-year time frame. See appendix I for more information on this category.

Pregnancy-related death, as defined in statute, is the death of a woman while pregnant or within 1 year of the end of a pregnancy— regardless of the outcome, duration or site of the pregnancy—from any cause related to or aggravated by the pregnancy or its management, but not from accidental or incidental causes. 42 U.S.C. § 247b-12(e)(3).

[a]According to CDC officials, there was a spike in pregnancy-related deaths due to infection in 2009 due to the H1N1 influenza epidemic.

Figure 4. Leading Causes of Pregnancy-Related Deaths, 2007-2016.

---

[26] E. E. Petersen, N. L. Davis, D. Goodman, et al. "Racial/Ethnic Disparities in Pregnancy-Related Deaths—United States, 2007–2016." *Morbidity and Mortality Weekly Report*, vol. 68, no. 35 (2019).

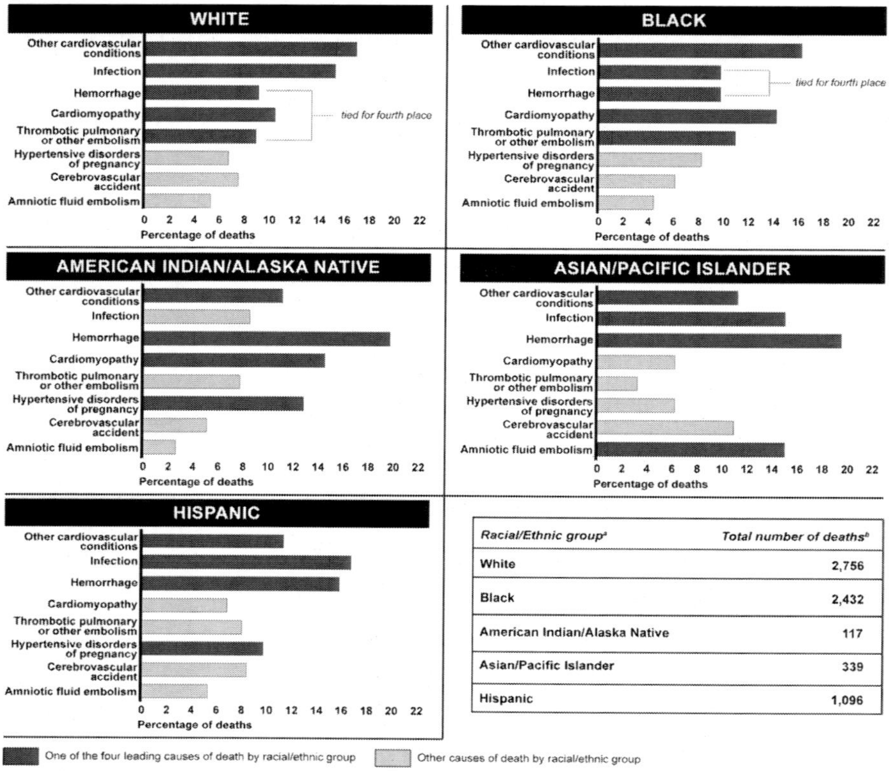

Racial/Ethnic group[a]	*Total number of deaths*[b]
White	2,756
Black	2,432
American Indian/Alaska Native	117
Asian/Pacific Islander	339
Hispanic	1,096

Source: GAO analysis of Centers for Control and prevention Pregnancy Mortality Surveillance System data. GAO-20-248. Notes: "Other cardiovascular conditions" includes conditions that are not reported separately as cardiomyopathy—when the normal muscle in the heart thicken, stiffen, thin out, or fill with substances the body produces that do not belong in the heart muscle, or cerebrovascular accidents—also known as stroke. In multiple CDC publications of Pregnancy Mortality Surveillance System data, "other non- cardiovascular medical conditions" is a leading cause of pregnancy-related deaths. GAO did not include this category in the figure because the category is composed of more than 10 diverse conditions, including cancer, autoimmune disease, and gastrointestinal disorders, among others, that each represent less than 3 percent of all pregnancy-related deaths for the 10-year time frame. See appendix I for more information on this category. Pregnancy-related death, as defined in statute, is the death of a woman while pregnant or within 1 year of the end of a pregnancy— regardless of the outcome, duration or site of the pregnancy—from any cause related to or aggravated by the pregnancy or its management, but not from accidental or incidental causes. 42 U.S.C. § 247b-12(e)(3). [a]White, black, American Indian/Alaska Native and Asian/Pacific Islander women were non-Hispanic. Hispanic women might be of any race. [b]From 2007 through 2016, there were 25 pregnancy-related deaths where race/ethnicity was unknown that were not included in our analyses.

Figure 5. Leading Causes of Pregnancy-Related Deaths by Racial/Ethnic Group, 2007-2016.

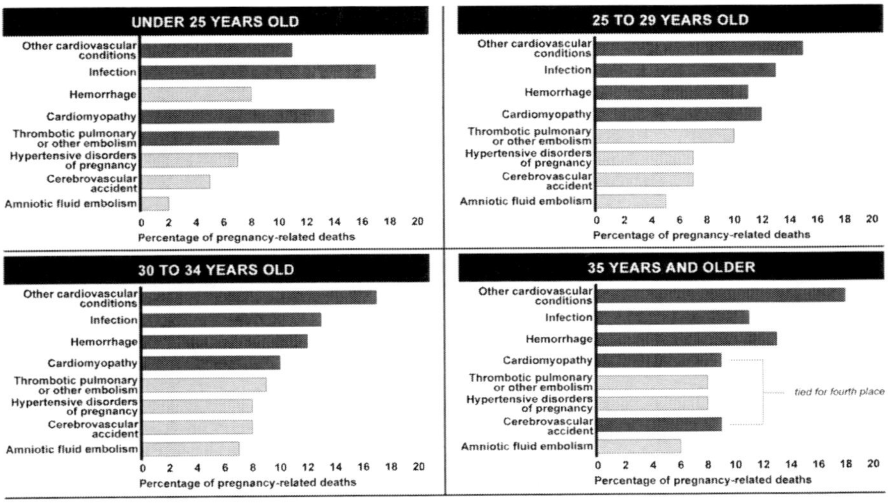

Age group	*Total number of deaths*[a]
Under 25 years old	1,501
25-29 years old	1,531
30-34 years old	1,602
35 years and older	2,129

One of the four leading causes of death by age group   Other causes of death by age group

Source: GAO analysis of Centers for Control and prevention Pregnancy Mortality Surveillance System data. GAO-20-248.

Notes: "Other cardiovascular conditions" includes conditions that are not reported separately as cardiomyopathy—when the normal muscle in the heart thicken, stiffen, thin out, or fill with substances the body produces that do not belong in the heart muscle, or cerebrovascular accidents—also known as stroke..

In multiple CDC publications of Pregnancy Mortality Surveillance System data, "other non-cardiovascular medical conditions" is a leading cause of pregnancy-related deaths. GAO did not include this category in the figure because the category is composed of more than 10 diverse conditions, including cancer, autoimmune disease, and gastrointestinal disorders, among others, that each represent less than 3 percent of all pregnancy-related deaths for the 10-year time frame. See appendix I for more information on this category.

Pregnancy-related death, as defined in statute, is the death of a woman while pregnant or within 1 year of the end of a pregnancy— regardless of the outcome, duration or site of the pregnancy—from any cause related to or aggravated by the pregnancy or its management, but not from accidental or incidental causes. 42 U.S.C. § 247b-12(e)(3).

[a]From 2007 through 2016, there were two pregnancy-related deaths where age was unknown that were not included in our analyses.

Figure 6. Leading Causes of Pregnancy-Related Deaths by Age Group, 2007-2016.

Leading causes of pregnancy-related deaths also differed by the age of the woman, as indicated by Figure 6. Specifically, the leading cause for women under 25 was infection, while for all other women the leading cause was other cardiovascular conditions. In a 2017 article, the authors noted that maternal morbidity and mortality rates increase with advanced maternal age, due in part to increased prevalence of chronic conditions (e.g., hypertension, diabetes, and chronic heart disease.).[27] This may help explain the variation in the rate of pregnancy-related deaths among women of different ages.

Most Pregnancy-Related Deaths Occurred within 42 Days of the End of Pregnancy, while Specific Causes of Death Varied Depending on When the Death Occurred

Our analysis of CDC's PMSS data shows that from 2011 through 2016, most pregnancy-related deaths occurred between 0 and 42 days postpartum—meaning that they occurred either on the day of delivery or end of pregnancy up to 42 days after pregnancy. (See Figure 7). According to CDC officials, understanding the timing of pregnancy-related deaths is important for prioritizing intervention strategies. The officials noted that deaths resulting from cardiomyopathy can occur months after pregnancy but can also be prevented with appropriate interventions. In particular, the American College of Obstetricians and Gynecologists published guidance for managing pregnancy and heart disease that noted that complications are frequently encountered in the days, weeks, and months after delivery in women with known cardiovascular disease and in those with latent cardiovascular disease. Women with multiple risk factors for

---

[27] N. L. Davis, D. L. Hoyert, D. A. Goodman, et al. "Contribution of maternal age and pregnancy checkbox on maternal mortality ratios in the United States, 1978-2012", *American Journal of Obstetrics & Gynecology, (*2017) 352.e1-7.

cardiovascular disease may be particularly at risk of manifesting symptoms for the first time during their postpartum course.[28]

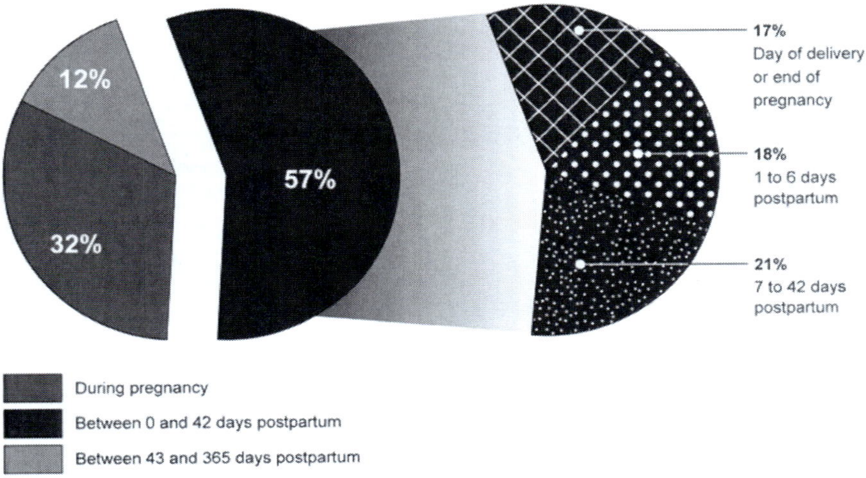

Source: GAO analysis of Centers for Control and prevention Pregnancy Mortality Surveillance System data. GAO-20-248.

Notes: Pregnancy-related death, as defined in statute, is the death of a woman while pregnant or within 1 year of the end of a pregnancy— regardless of the outcome, duration or site of the pregnancy— from any cause related to or aggravated by the pregnancy or its management, but not from accidental or incidental causes. 42 U.S.C. § 247b-12(e)(3).

Percentages in this graphic do not total 100 due to rounding.

According to CDC officials, data on the timing of death relative to pregnancy are only available for 2011-2016, and the specific timing of death is known for almost 88 percent (or 3,573) of the pregnancy-related deaths from this time.

Figure 7. Pregnancy-Related Deaths by Timing of Death Relative to Pregnancy, 2011-2016.

CDC's data show that the leading causes of pregnancy-related death varied depending on when the death occurred. For example, over the period 2011-2016, hemorrhage and amniotic fluid embolism were leading causes of pregnancy-related deaths on the day of delivery or the end of pregnancy, while cardiomyopathy was the leading cause of pregnancy-related deaths between 43 and 365 days postpartum. (See Figure 8)

---

28 American College of Obstetricians and Gynecologists. "ACOG Practice Bulletin No. 212: Pregnancy and Heart Disease." *Obstetrics & Gynecology*, vol. 133, no. 5 (2019), e320- 356.

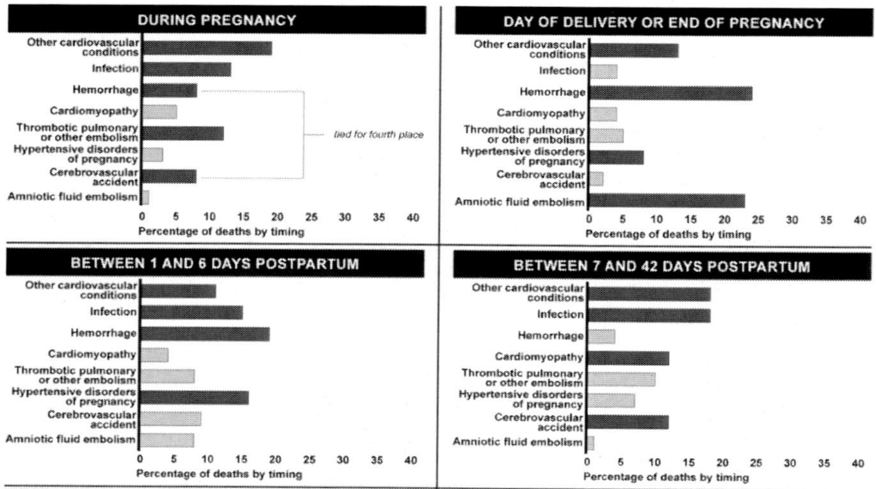

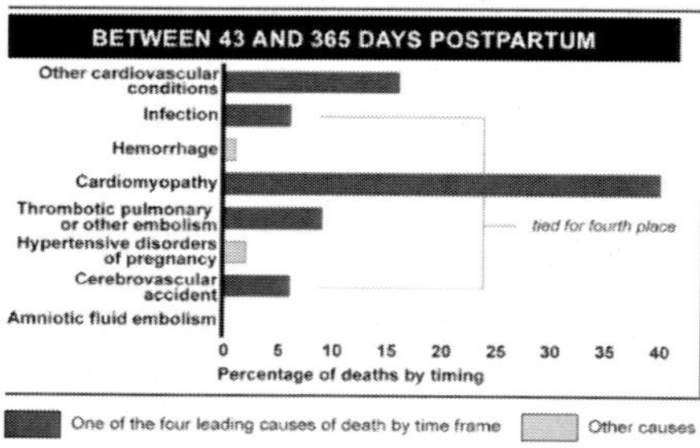

Time frame	Total number of deaths[a]
During pregnancy	1,133
Day of delivery or end of pregnancy	603
Between 1 and 6 days postpartum	651
Between 7 and 42 days postpartum	767
Between 43 and 365 days postpartum	419

Source: GAO analysis of Centers for Control and prevention Pregnancy Mortality Surveillance System data. GAO-20-248.

Notes: "Other cardiovascular conditions" includes conditions that are not reported separately as cardiomyopathy—when the normal muscles in the heart thicken, stiffen, thin out, or fill with substances the body produces that do not belong in the heart muscle, or cerebrovascular accidents— also known as stroke. In multiple CDC publications of Pregnancy Mortality Surveillance System data, "other non- cardiovascular medical conditions" is a leading cause of pregnancy-related deaths. GAO did not include this category in the figure because the category is composed of more than 10 diverse conditions, including cancer, autoimmune disease, and gastrointestinal disorders, among others, that each represent less than 3 percent of all pregnancy-related deaths for the 10-year time frame. See appendix I for more information on this category.

Pregnancy-related death, as defined in statute, is the death of a woman while pregnant or within 1 year of the end of a pregnancy— regardless of the outcome, duration or site of the pregnancy—from any cause related to or aggravated by the pregnancy or its management, but not from accidental or incidental causes. 42 U.S.C. § 247b-12(e)(3).

[a]According to CDC officials, data on the timing of death relative to pregnancy are only available for 2011-2016, and the specific timing of death is known for almost 88 percent (or 3,573) of the pregnancy-related deaths from this time.

Figure 8. Leading Causes of Pregnancy-Related Deaths by Timing of Death Relative to Pregnancy, 2011-2016.

A recent article on pregnancy-related deaths stated that multiple factors contribute to pregnancy-related deaths during pregnancy, labor and delivery, and the postpartum period.

Further, the article notes that no single intervention strategy is sufficient, and reducing these deaths requires reviewing and learning from each death, improving women's health, and reducing social inequities across the life span, as well as ensuring quality care for pregnant and postpartum women, according to the article.[29] See appendix II for supplemental data on pregnancy-related deaths.

HHS Funds Multiple Ongoing Efforts Focused on Reducing Pregnancy-Related Deaths

HHS has 13 ongoing funding efforts aimed at reducing pregnancy-related deaths, one of which is exclusively focused on reducing pregnancy-related deaths, while the others have additional focus areas, such as improving infant health.[30] (See appendix III for details on each of the 13 efforts and appendix IV for additional details on HRSA- and NIH-funded research.) Below are summaries of two of the key funding efforts, one of which is exclusively focused on reducing maternal mortality and the other involves annual awards to 59 states and jurisdictions:

- Preventing Maternal Deaths: Supporting Maternal Mortality Review Committees Cooperative Agreements. Under these cooperative agreements, CDC is providing funding to state agencies and organizations that coordinate and manage MMRCs.[31]

---

[29] E. E. Petersen, N. L. Davis, D. Goodman, et al. "Vital Signs: Pregnancy-Related Deaths, United States, 2011–2015, and Strategies for Prevention, 13 States, 2013–2017." *Morbidity and Mortality Weekly Report (MMWR)*, vol. 68, no. 18 (2019):423–429.

[30] Two of these efforts are not discrete funding opportunities, but rather a variety of research funding opportunities offered by HRSA and NIH.

[31] Previously, in December 2015, CDC, the CDC Foundation, and the Association of Maternal and Child Health Programs partnered to launch the Building U.S. Capacity to Review and Prevent Maternal Deaths initiative to address barriers that MMRCs face in achieving full functionality and sustainability. Merck, on behalf of its Merck for Mothers Program, funded

As previously mentioned, MMRCs systematically and comprehensively review pregnancy-related deaths in order to identify prevention opportunities.[32] Funding recipients will identify and review deaths within 1 year of death and enter clinical and non-clinical data and committee decisions in MMRIA—a standardized data system managed by CDC—within 2 years of death. As part of the agreement, recipients—in coordination with CDC—analyze data and share findings with stakeholders, such as clinicians, to inform policy and prevention strategies to reduce pregnancy-related deaths, such as screening procedures. According to CDC officials, in August 2019, CDC awarded these 5-year cooperative agreements to 24 recipients covering 25 states.[33] Recipients received different amounts ranging from $150,000 to over $550,000 in the first year to support their MMRC. CDC anticipates awarding a similar level of funding for the 5- year period of performance.

- Maternal and Child Health (MCH) Services Block Grant Program. HRSA provides funding through this program to 59 states and jurisdictions to improve maternal and child health.[34] According to agency officials, many recipients reported using their MCH Services Block Grant funding to help support or complement other federal initiatives, such as an MMRC, a Perinatal Quality Collaborative (PQC), and Alliance for Innovation on Maternal

the initiative through an agreement with CDC Foundation. In FY 2019, Congress provided CDC funding for CDC's work with MMRCs.

[32] MMRCs are multidisciplinary committees at the state and jurisdiction-level, including doctors, nurses, social workers, researchers, and others, that systematically and comprehensively review clinical and non-clinical information about pregnancy-related deaths to develop recommended strategies for preventing future deaths.

[33] According to CDC, the recipients include Alaska, Arizona, California, Colorado, Connecticut, Delaware, Illinois, Indiana, Kansas, Louisiana, Mississippi, Missouri, New Hampshire, New Jersey, New Mexico, New York, North Carolina, Ohio, Pennsylvania, Tennessee, Texas, Utah, Washington, and Wisconsin. Additionally, Utah's award includes a subcontract to support review of deaths in Wyoming.

[34] HRSA, an agency within HHS, is the primary agency for improving health care for those who are geographically isolated, and/or economically or medically vulnerable, such as pregnant women and mothers.

Health (AIM) maternal safety bundles.[35] For example, according to HRSA officials, in fiscal year 2018, 38 recipients self-reported that the block grant partially or fully funded their MMRCs, and additional states and jurisdictions reported using block grant support for planning activities to begin development of their MMRC. Further, states and jurisdictions cited PQCs, networks of multidisciplinary teams that work to improve measurable outcomes for maternal and infant health, in their block grant narrative.[36] Additionally, implementation of a HRSA-supported AIM maternal safety bundle, sets of actionable, evidence-based practices for improving maternal outcomes was cited.[37] (Appendix III includes more information on funding for PQCs and AIM maternal safety bundles.) Our review of HRSA documentation shows that in fiscal year 2017, total federal expenditures for the block grant program were about $540 million for women and children covered by the program, and expenditures for services for pregnant women from all sources—federal funds, as well as state, local, program income, and other funds—was about $300 million.[38]

---

[35] CDC also provides funds for MMRCs and PQCs through cooperative agreements, and HRSA also provides funds for AIM maternal safety bundles through cooperative agreements.

[36] State PQCs are networks of multidisciplinary teams that work to improve measurable outcomes for maternal and infant health by advancing evidence-informed clinical practices using quality improvement principles. PQCs work with clinical teams, experts, and stakeholders, including patients and families, to disseminate best practices and optimize resources to improve perinatal care and outcomes.

[37] AIM maternal safety bundles are sets of evidence-based practices that when implemented collectively and reliably in the delivery setting may improve patient outcomes and may reduce maternal mortality and severe maternal morbidity.

[38] These block grants may be used by states "to provide and to assure mothers and children (in particular those with low income or with limited availability of health services) access to quality maternal and child health services," among other things. 42 U.S.C. §701(a)(1)(A). States determine the actual services provided under the block grant. For example, a state may provide medical services in sectors where public and private health insurers offer limited coverage options, such as coverage for dental and durable medical equipment (e.g., wheelchairs and oxygen equipment).

State Participation in the Alliance for Innovation on Maternal Health (AIM) Initiative

According to the American College of Obstetrics and Gynecology, as of June 2019, 26 states were enrolled in the AIM initiative. The AIM initiative, funded by the Health Resources and Services Administration, engages provider organizations, state-based public health systems, consumer groups and others in a national partnership to assist state- based teams in implementing evidence-based maternal safety bundles.

Ten of the 26 states joined in the last year and are beginning to implement maternal safety bundles and collect data. Five of these bundles are being implemented by one or more states. Bundle topics: Maternal Venous Thromboembolism, Postpartum Care Basics for Maternal Safety: From Birth to Comprehensive Postpartum Visit, Obstetric Care for Women with Opioid Use Disorder, Obstetric Hemorrhage, Reduction of Peripartum Racial/Ethnic Disparities, Safe Reduction of Primary Cesarean Birth, Severe Hypertension in Pregnancy, and Postpartum Care Basics for Maternal Safety: Transition from Maternity to Well Woman Care.

Source: American College of Obstetricians and Gynecologists. | GAO-20-248.

According to officials we interviewed in five selected states, they use these two efforts—MMRC findings and MCH block grant funding—and other efforts collectively to address pregnancy-related deaths. For example, according to Georgia officials, Georgia's PQC received funding from CDC and implemented the AIM obstetric hemorrhage maternal safety bundle in 2018 based on the state's MMRC finding that hemorrhage was a leading cause of pregnancy-related deaths in Georgia. According to officials, Georgia's MMRC was funded primarily through the MCH Services Block Grant. Similarly, according to Maryland officials, Maryland's PQC oversees implementation of the state's AIM initiative.

Officials we interviewed from three of the five selected states said that the AIM initiative had an immediate or the largest effect on addressing maternal mortality in their state. Officials from the other two states said they could not identify which efforts had the largest or most immediate effect on addressing maternal mortality. Officials from one state noted the importance of their collaborative approach and the other noted that there is no one contributing factor for maternal mortality. See appendix V for more information about how the selected states we interviewed are using these funding efforts.

Indian Health Service (IHS) Implementation of Alliance for Innovation on Maternal Health (AIM) Maternal Safety Bundles

In 2017, IHS's leadership released a request that IHS federal hospitals that provide inpatient obstetric care implement at least one maternal safety bundle—sets of evidence- based practices that when implemented collectively and reliably in the delivery setting may improve patient outcomes and reduce maternal mortality and severe maternal morbidity. According to IHS, since 2014, IHS has had phased implementation of the bundles in federal hospitals that provide inpatient obstetric care.

Officials said that for many facilities, Obstetric Hemorrhage was the first bundle implemented. Others have also been implemented, such as the Severe Hypertension in Pregnancy bundle, and the Obstetric Care for Women with Opioid Use Disorder bundle.

Source: Indian Health Service. | GAO-20-248.

All five states also mentioned beginning or continuing to address racial/ethnic or other health disparities with block grant funding, through their MMRCs, or other efforts. For example, officials in one state said they use block grant funding to support its Black Infant Health Program, which helps address maternal morbidity and mortality of black mothers in the late maternal period. Additionally, two of the HHS funding efforts awarded in fiscal year 2019 have outcomes related to decreasing racial and ethnic disparities in maternal mortality: the Alliance for Innovation on Maternal Health Community Care Initiative and the State Maternal Health Innovation Program.

In addition to those efforts that are exclusive to maternal mortality or have a focus on maternal mortality, HHS agencies have other funding efforts that may reduce maternal mortality by improving maternal health. For example, agency officials also identified the following:

- HRSA's Maternal, Infant, and Early Childhood Home Visiting Program supports voluntary, evidence-based home visiting services for at-risk pregnant women and parents with children up to kindergarten entry. Our review of agency documentation shows that in fiscal year 2019, HRSA awarded about $351 million in funding to 56 states, territories, and nonprofit organizations to support communities in providing voluntary evidence-based home visiting services through the Maternal, Infant, and Early Childhood Home Visiting Program.
- The Substance Abuse and Mental Health Services Administration, which is responsible for leading public health efforts to advance the behavioral health of the nation and reducing the impact of substance abuse and mental illness on America's communities. The agency funds two programs that provide grants to public and private nonprofit entities and state substance abuse agencies for substance use disorder treatment and recovery services for pregnant and postpartum women. Our review of agency documentation and interviews with agency officials shows that from fiscal year 2017 through 2019, the Substance Abuse and Mental Health Services Administration awarded 41 Services Grant Program for Residential Treatment for Pregnant and Postpartum Women and six State Pilot Grant Program for Treatment for Pregnant and Postpartum Women grants.
- The Centers for Medicare & Medicaid Services, which administers the Medicare and Medicaid programs, developed the Maternal Opioid Misuse Model. Through this model, state Medicaid agencies will coordinate with care-delivery partners to test whether payments for evidence-based, coordinated care delivery improve outcomes and reduce costs for pregnant and postpartum Medicaid beneficiaries with opioid use disorder and their infants. According to agency officials, funding for cooperative agreements with 10 state Medicaid agencies began in January 2020.

AGENCY COMMENTS

We provided a draft of this chapter to HHS. HHS provided technical comments, which we incorporated as appropriate.

As agreed with your offices, unless you publicly announce the contents of this chapter earlier, we plan no further distribution until 30 days from the report date. At that time, we will send copies of this chapter to the Secretary of HHS, and appropriate congressional committees.

Mary Denigan-Macauley
Director, Health Care

List of Requesters

The Honorable Patty Murray
Ranking Member
Committee on Health, Education, Labor, and Pensions
United States Senate

The Honorable Tammy Baldwin
United States Senate

The Honorable Cory A. Booker
United States Senate

The Honorable Benjamin L. Cardin
United States Senate

The Honorable Thomas R. Carper
United States Senate

The Honorable Richard J. Durbin
United States Senate

The Honorable Kirsten Gillibrand
United States Senate

The Honorable Kamala D. Harris
United States Senate

The Honorable Debbie Stabenow
United States Senate

The Honorable Elizabeth Warren
United States Senate

The Honorable Ron Wyden
United States Senate

APPENDIX I: PREGNANCY MORTALITY SURVEILLANCE SYSTEM CAUSE OF DEATH CATEGORIES

In 1986, the Centers for Disease Control and Prevention (CDC) initiated national surveillance of pregnancy-related deaths in the Pregnancy Mortality Surveillance System (PMSS) because more clinical information was needed to fill data gaps about causes of these deaths. A pregnancy-related death, as defined in statute, is the death of a woman while pregnant or within 1 year of the end of a pregnancy—regardless of the outcome, duration or site of the pregnancy—from any cause related to or aggravated by the pregnancy or its management, but not from accidental or incidental causes.[39]

[39] 42 U.S.C. § 247b-12(e)(3).

Table 1. Cause of Pregnancy-Related Deaths Category Information and Related Statistics, 2007 through 2016

Cause of Death Category		
Other cardiovascular conditions (accounts for about 15 percent of deaths)	Examples of associated conditions:	Other cardiovascular conditions include coronary artery disease (plaque buildup in the walls of the arteries that supply blood to the heart and other parts of the body), pulmonary hypertension (high blood pressure in the blood vessels that carry blood to the lungs), and valvular heart disease (damage to or a defect in one of the four heart valves), among others
	Leading cause of death for:	Non-Hispanic black women (about 16 percent of deaths for this racial group) and non-Hispanic white women (about 17 percent of deaths for this racial group)
	Most common time frame:[a]	During pregnancy (about 38 percent of these deaths from other cardiovascular conditions)
	Most common age group affected:	Women 35 years and older (about 37 percent of deaths from other cardiovascular conditions)
Infection (accounts for about 13 percent of deaths)	Examples of associated conditions:	Infection includes conditions, such as sepsis (when the body has an extreme response to an infection that can rapidly lead to tissue damage, organ failure, and death), urinary tract infections (an infection in any part of your urinary system—kidneys, ureters, bladder and urethra), and others, such as influenza.
	Leading cause of death for:	Hispanic women (about 17 percent of deaths for this racial group)
	Most common time frame:[a]	During pregnancy (about 33 percent of deaths from infection) or between 7 and 42 days postpartum (about 33 percent of deaths from infection)
	Most common age group affected:	Women under 25 years old (about 29 percent of deaths from infection)
Cardiomyopathy (accounts for about 11 percent of deaths)	Examples of associated conditions:	Cardiomyopathy occurs when the normal muscle in the heart thicken, stiffen, thin out, or fill with substances the body produces that do not belong in the heart muscle.
	Leading cause of death for:	No racial/ethnic groups
	Most common time frame:[a]	Between 43 and 365 days postpartum (about 45 percent of deaths from cardiomyopathy)
	Most common age group affected:	Women under 25 years old (about 29 percent of deaths from cardiomyopathy)

Table 1. (Continued)

Cause of Death Category		
Hemorrhage (accounts for about 11 percent of deaths)	Examples of associated conditions:	Hemorrhage includes placental abruption (when the placenta partially or completely separates from the inner wall of the uterus before delivery), ruptured ectopic pregnancy (when a fertilized egg implants outside of the uterus, such as in a fallopian tube, and ruptures as it grows), and hemorrhage due to retained placenta (generally when the placenta is not expelled within 30 minutes of delivery of the infant).
	Leading cause of death for:	Non-Hispanic American Indian/Alaska Native women (about 20 percent of deaths for this racial group) and non-Hispanic Asian/Pacific Islander women (about 20 percent of deaths for this racial group)
	Most common time frame:[a]	Day of delivery or the end of pregnancy (about 38 percent of deaths from hemorrhage)
	Most common age group affected:	Women 35 years and older (about 36 percent of deaths from hemorrhage)
Thrombotic pulmonary or other embolism (accounts for about 9 percent of deaths)	Examples of associated conditions:	Thrombotic, pulmonary, or other embolisms include deep vein thrombosis (when a blood clot forms in a deep vein, usually in the lower leg, thigh, or pelvis), and pulmonary embolism (when a clot breaks loose and travels through the bloodstream to the lungs).
	Leading cause of death for:	No racial/ethnic groups
	Most common time frame:[a]	During pregnancy (about 40 percent of deaths from a thrombotic embolism)
	Most common age group affected:	Women 35 years and older (about 28 percent of deaths from a thrombotic embolism)
Hypertensive disorders of pregnancy (accounts for about 8 percent of deaths)	Examples of associated conditions:	Hypertensive disorders of pregnancy include conditions, such as preeclampsia (high blood pressure during pregnancy or postpartum and other organ damage (e.g., liver or kidney damage) and eclampsia (the new onset of seizures or coma in a pregnant woman with preeclampsia).
	Leading cause of death for:	No racial/ethnic groups

Cause of Death Category		
	Most common time frame:[a]	Between 1 and 6 days postpartum (about 42 percent of deaths from hypertensive disorders of pregnancy)
	Most common age group affected:	Women 35 years and older (about 33 percent of deaths from hypertensive disorders of pregnancy)
Cerebrovascular accidents (accounts about 7 percent of deaths)	Examples of associated conditions:	Cerebrovascular accidents, also known as stroke, include ischemic stroke when an artery that supplies blood to the brain is blocked and part of the brain goes without blood for too long or hemorrhagic stroke when an artery in the brain leaks blood or ruptures. An aneurysm is an example of condition that can cause a hemorrhagic stroke.
	Leading cause of death for:	No racial/ethnic groups
	Most common time frame:[a]	Between 7 and 42 days postpartum (about 33 percent of deaths from cerebrovascular accidents)
	Most common age group affected:	Women 35 and older (about 37 percent of deaths from cerebrovascular accidents)
Unknown (accounts for about 6 percent of deaths)	Examples of associated conditions:	Officials told us that unknown includes deaths where pregnancy complications, obstetric complications, among others were listed as the cause of death on the death certificate.
	Leading cause of death for:	No racial/ethnic groups
	Most common time frame:[a]	During pregnancy (about 41 percent of deaths from an unknown cause)
	Most common age group affected:	Women 35 and older (about 34 percent of deaths from an unknown cause)
Amniotic fluid embolism (accounts for about 5 percent of deaths) Cause of Death Category	Examples of associated conditions:	Amniotic fluid embolism occurs when amniotic fluid enters into the maternal circulation.
	Leading cause of death for:	No racial/ethnic groups
	Most common time frame:a	Day of delivery or end of pregnancy (about 64 percent of deaths from an amniotic fluid embolism)
	Most common age group affected:	Women 35 and older (about 38 percent of deaths from an amniotic fluid embolism)

Table 1. (Continued)

Cause of Death Category		
Anesthesia- complications (accounts less than 1 percent of deaths)	Examples of associated conditions:	Anesthesia complications include aspiration pneumonia due to anesthesia, which involves when there is swelling or an infection of the lungs or large airways.
	Leading cause of death for:	No racial/ethnic groups
	Most common time frame:[a]	Day of delivery or end of pregnancy (about 33 percent of deaths from anesthesia complications) and between 1 and 6 days postpartum (about 33 percent of deaths from anesthesia complications)
	Most common age group affected:	Women 30 to 34 years old (about 33 percent of deaths from anesthesia complications)
Other non- cardiovascular medical conditions (accounts for about 13 percent of deaths)	Examples of associated conditions:	Other non-cardiovascular medical conditions includes a range of conditions, such as: • Hematologic, such as sickle cell disease, a group of inherited red blood cell disorders. • Collagen vascular/autoimmune diseases, such as systemic lupus erythematosus —the most common type of lupus—in which the immune system attacks its own tissues, causing widespread inflammation and tissue damage in the affected organs, such as lungs, kidneys, and blood vessels. • Immune deficiency problems, such as human immunodeficiency virus infection, which interferes with your body's ability to fight the organisms that cause disease and over time can weaken the immune system and result in acquired immunodeficiency syndrome. • Cancer, such as gestational trophoblastic disease, which is a group of rare tumors that involve abnormal growth of cells inside a woman's uterus. • Pulmonary conditions, such as cystic fibrosis, which is an inherited disease characterized by the buildup of thick, sticky mucus that can damage many of the body's organs and commonly includes progressive damage to the respiratory system and chronic digestive system problems. • Neurologic conditions, such as epilepsy/seizure disorder, which is a brain disorder that

Cause of Death Category		
		• causes repeated seizures and can cause brief changes in how a person behaves, thinks, or feels. • Renal disease, such as chronic kidney failure, which is the gradual loss of kidney function and when it reaches an advanced stage, dangerous levels of fluid, electrolytes and wastes can build up in your body. • Endocrine/metabolic, such as obesity, which is a complex disease involving an excessive amount of body fat and increases your risk of other diseases and health problems, such as heart disease, diabetes, high blood pressure and certain cancers. • Gastrointestinal disorders, such as Crohn's disease, which is an inflammatory bowel disease that can be painful and debilitating, and sometimes may lead to life-threatening complications.
Leading cause of death for:		No racial/ethnic group
Most common time frame:[a]		During pregnancy (about 53 percent of deaths from other non-cardiovascular medical conditions)
Most common age group affected:		Women under 25 years old (about 30 percent of deaths from other non- cardiovascular medical conditions)

Source: GAO analysis of Pregnancy Mortality Surveillance System data, Department of Health and Human Services documents and officials, and other documents. | GAO-20-248.

[a]According to CDC officials, data on the timing of death relative to pregnancy are only available from 2011 through 2016, and the specific timing of death is known for almost 88 percent (or 3,573)of the pregnancy-related deaths from this time.

As of September 2019, CDC used 11 categories when coding the cause of death for pregnancy-related deaths in PMSS, and 2016 data were the most recent data available. From 2007 through 2016, there were 6,765 pregnancy-related deaths, according to PMSS data. See table below for information on the 11 cause of pregnancy-related death categories, including PMSS data on leading causes, most common time frame, and most common age group affected.

APPENDIX II: SUPPLEMENTAL DATA ON PREGNANCY-RELATED DEATHS

The following tables include supplemental data on pregnancy-related deaths by racial/ethnic and age groups

Table 2. Percentage of Pregnancy-Related Deaths by Racial/Ethnic Group for Each Age Range, 2007-2016

Age range				
Racial/Ethnic group[a]	Percentage of women under 25 years old	Percentage of women 25-29 years old	Percentage of women 30-34 years old	Percentage of women 35 years and older
White women (n = 2,756)	21	22	25	33
Black women (n = 2,431)	26	24	22	29
American Indian/Alaska Native	22	23	23	32
Asian/Pacific Islander, women	7	19	34	40
Hispanic women (n = 1,096)	23	23	23	31
All women (n = 6,739)[b]	22	23	24	31

Source: GAO analysis of Pregnancy Mortality Surveillance System data. | GAO-20-248.

Note: Pregnancy-related death, as defined in statute, is the death of a woman while pregnant or within 1 year of the end of a pregnancy— regardless of the outcome, duration or site of the pregnancy— from any cause related to or aggravated by the pregnancy or its management, but not from accidental or incidental causes. 42 U.S.C. § 247b-12(e)(3).

Percentages do not always add to 100 due to rounding.

[a]White, black, American Indian/Alaska Native and Asian/Pacific Islander women were non-Hispanic. Hispanic women might be of any race.

[b]From 2007 through 2016, there were 26 pregnancy-related deaths where race/ethnicity or age was unknown that were not included in our analyses.

Table 3. Percentage of Pregnancy-Related Deaths by Racial/Ethnic Group for Each Time Frame Relative to Pregnancy, 2011- 2016

Racial/Ethnic group[a]	**Percentage of**				
	During pregnancy	Between 0 and 42 days postpartum			Between 43 and 365 days postpartum
		Day of delivery or the end of pregnancy	Between 1 and 6 days postpartum	Between 7 and 42 days postpartum	
White women (n = 1,493)	34	16	18	21	11
Black women (n = 1,278)	33	15	15	23	14
American Indian/Alaska Native women (n = 56)	30	14	23	16	16
Asian/Pacific Islander women (n = 203)	16	33	28	14	9
Hispanic women (n = 536)	26	18	23	23	10
All women (n = 3,566)[b]	32	17	18	21	12

Source: GAO analysis of Pregnancy Mortality Surveillance System data | GAO-20-248.

Note: Pregnancy-related death, as defined in statute, is the death of a woman while pregnant or within 1 year of the end of a pregnancy— regardless of the outcome, duration or site of the pregnancy— from any cause related to or aggravated by the pregnancy or its management, but not from accidental or incidental causes. 42 U.S.C. § 247b-12(e)(3).

Percentages do not always add to 100 due to rounding.

[a]White, black, American Indian/Alaska Native and Asian/Pacific Islander women were non-Hispanic. Hispanic women might be of any race.

[b]According to CDC officials, data on the timing of death relative to pregnancy are only available for 2011-2016, and the specific timing of death is known for almost 88 percent (or 3,573) of the pregnancy-related deaths from this time. Of the deaths with available timing information, there were seven pregnancy-related deaths where the race/ethnicity was unknown that were not included in this analysis.

Table 4. Percentage of Pregnancy-Related Deaths by Age Group for Each Time Frame Relative to Pregnancy, 2011-2016

Age group	Percentage of pregnancy-related deaths				
	During pregnancy	Between 0 and 42 days postpartum			Between 43 and 365 days
		Day of delivery or the end of pregnancy	Between 1 and 6 days postpartum	Between 7 and 42 days postpartum	
Women under 25 years old (n = 743)	32	14	15	22	16
Women 25-29 years old (n = 808)	29	16	18	25	12
Women 30-34 years old (n = 855)	27	20	21	22	10
Women 35 years and older (n = 1,167)	36	17	18	19	10
All women (n = 3,573)[a]	32	17	18	21	12

Source: GAO analysis of Pregnancy Mortality Surveillance System data. | GAO-20-248.

Note: Pregnancy-related death, as defined in statute, is the death of a woman while pregnant or within 1 year of the end of a pregnancy— regardless of the outcome, duration or site of the pregnancy— from any cause related to or aggravated by the pregnancy or its management, but not from accidental or incidental causes. 42 U.S.C. § 247b-12(e)(3).

Percentages do not always add to 100 due to rounding.

[a]According to CDC officials, data on the timing of death relative to pregnancy are only available for 2011-2016, and the specific timing of death is known for almost 88 percent (or 3,573) of the pregnancy-related deaths from this time.

Appendix III: Ongoing Department of Health and Human Services Funding Efforts to Reduce Pregnancy-Related Deaths

As of September 2019, the Department of Health and Human Services was providing funding for 13 efforts with a stated outcome, goal, or focus on reducing pregnancy-related deaths. One of the these—Supporting Maternal Mortality Review Committees—is funded by CDC and has an exclusive focus on reducing deaths of the women during pregnancy or up to 1 year of pregnancy, while the other 12 have additional focus areas, such as improving infant health. Two of these efforts are not discrete funding opportunities, but rather a variety of research funding opportunities offered by the Health Resources and Services Administration and the National Institutes of Health. Table 5 lists the 13 efforts, their current awards, funding, purpose, and examples of goals or research.

Table 5. Ongoing Department of Health and Human Services (HHS) Funding Efforts with a Focus on Pregnancy-Related Deaths

Ongoing HHS Funding Opportunities	**Centers for Disease Control and Prevention (CDC)**
Preventing Maternal Deaths: Supporting Maternal Mortality Review Committees (MMRC)	*Funding details*: In 2019, CDC awarded 24 5-year cooperative agreements; recipients received between \$150,000 and over \$550,000 in funding each year for a total funding amount of about \$8.4 million across all awardees for fiscal year 2019. *Purpose:* Supports MMRC's ability to collect the most detailed, complete data on causes and circumstances surrounding pregnancy-related deaths to develop recommendations for prevention. This multidisciplinary approach encourages collaboration with clinical and non-clinical partnerships to improve quality of care and address social determinants of health to reduce health inequities. *Examples of goals:*[a] 1) Short-term outcome: timely, accurate, and standardized information available about deaths to women during pregnancy and the year after the end of pregnancy, including opportunities for prevention, within funded jurisdictions and across funded jurisdictions; and 2) long-term outcome: reduction in maternal complications of pregnancy.
State-based Perinatal Quality Collaboratives (PQC) Cooperative Agreements	*Funding details*: In 2017, CDC awarded 13 5-year cooperative agreements to states with up to \$200,000 in annual funding for a total funding amount of about \$2.6 million per year across all awardees. These states included New York – which had received funding in both in the 2011 and 2014 award cycles – New Jersey, Delaware, Florida, Georgia, Illinois, Louisiana, Massachusetts, Minnesota, Mississippi, Oregon, and Wisconsin. Previous award cycles in 2011 and 2014 provided funding to three and six states, respectively. *Purpose:* Supports states' ability to enhance the capacity of PQC—networks of multidisciplinary teams that work to improve measurable outcomes for maternal and infant health—in early stages of development by conducting quality improvement projects.

Table 5. (Continued)

Ongoing HHS Funding Opportunities	Centers for Disease Control and Prevention (CDC)
	These projects include reduction of maternal morbidity and mortality and reduction of medically unnecessary cesarean deliveries. *Examples of goals:*[a] 1) Short-term outcome: increased participation of hospitals throughout the state in the PQC; 2) intermediate outcome: service delivery improvements made statewide; and 3) long-term outcome: improvements in perinatal measures
National Network of Perinatal Quality Collaboratives Cooperative Agreement	*Funding details*: In 2017, CDC awarded a 5-year cooperative agreement to the National Institute for Children's Health Quality with about $228,000 in annual funding. *Purpose:* Supports PQCs nationwide (funded and unfunded) to improve care and programming related to maternal and infant health broadly including through promoting collaborative learning, through providing technical assistance in the use of rapid response data and quality improvement support, and through providing resources to states. *Examples of goals:*[a] 1) Short-term outcome: improved communication among PQCs across the country; 2) intermediate outcome: development and sustainment of more fully functioning PQCs across the country; and 3) long-term outcome: improvements in perinatal measures.
Stop the Clot, Spread the Word®	*Funding details*: In 2015, CDC awarded the National Blood Clot Alliance a cooperative agreement with about $365,045 in annual funding for 5 years for a total award amount of about $1.8 million. According to CDC, approximately $365,045 of the total amount awarded was applied to the campaign that specifically focuses on pregnancy and blood clots. *Purpose*: Supports national digital campaigns that provide information on the risk factors, signs, and symptoms of venous thromboembolism or blood clots, including one that focuses on pulmonary embolism or blood clots in the lungs—one of the most common causes of pregnancy-related deaths in the United States. *Examples of goals:*[a] 1) Increased knowledge and awareness of the signs, symptoms, and best treatments for venous thromboembolism by consumers and healthcare providers; and 2) increased adherence to venous thromboembolism treatment.
Health Resources and Services Administration (HRSA)	
Maternal and Child Health (MCH) Services Block Grants	*Funding details*: In fiscal year 2017, HRSA awarded block grants to 59 states and jurisdictions which had over $6 billion in expenditures of federal, state, local, and other funds for maternal and child health, with approximately $300 million of which were for services for pregnant women.
	Purpose: States use this funding to, among other things, support promotion of health and wellbeing before, during, and after pregnancy. Commonly cited activities supported or complemented by the block

Ongoing HHS Funding Opportunities	Centers for Disease Control and Prevention (CDC)
Maternal and Child Health (MCH) Services Block Grants	grants include other federal initiatives such as MMRCs, PQCs, and implementation of Alliance for Innovation on Maternal Health (AIM) maternal safety bundles. There are three levels of service in block grant programs that include direct services, enabling service, and public health services and systems.
	Examples of goals:[a] 1) National Outcome Measures which are longer-term measures, include Early Prenatal Care, Severe Maternal Morbidity, and Maternal Mortality, and 2) National Performance Measures, short term indicators that influence national outcome measures, related to women/maternal health include well-woman visits, low-risk cesarean deliveries, preventive dental visits during pregnancy, and smoking during pregnancy. Based on their identified priorities, each state or jurisdiction has to select at least one of these four national performance measures
Alliance for Innovation on Maternal Health (AIM) Cooperative Agreement	*Funding details*: In fiscal year 2018, HRSA awarded a 5-year cooperative agreement to the American College of Obstetricians and Gynecologists with $2 million in annual funding. According to the American College of Obstetricians and Gynecologists, the approved budget in the cooperative agreement provides states enrolling in AIM the opportunity to receive $26,000 in the state's initial year of membership. After the first year, states may receive up to $16,000 additional funding to further support implementation if necessary. Otherwise, AIM states receive $9,000 to support travel and bundle implementation support sessions. *Purpose*: Supports efforts to reduce maternal deaths and severe maternal morbidity by engaging provider organizations, state-based public health systems, consumer groups and other stakeholders in a national partnership to develop and implement evidence-based maternal safety bundles. *Examples of goals:*[a] 1) Facilitate widespread implementation of the current maternal safety bundles and/or resources; and 2) develop new maternal safety bundles and/or resources that address new topics in the quality and safety of maternity care practices.
Alliance for Innovation on Maternal Health (AIM) Community Care Initiative	*Funding details*: In fiscal year 2019, HRSA awarded a 5-year cooperative agreement to the National Healthy Start Association, Inc. with about $1.83 million in annual funding. *Purpose:* Supports the development and implementation of non-hospital focused maternal safety bundles within community-based organizations and outpatient clinical settings and builds upon the foundational work of the Alliance for Innovation on Maternal Health by addressing preventable maternal mortality and severe maternal morbidity among pregnant and postpartum women outside of hospital and birthing facility settings.

Table 5. (Continued)

Ongoing HHS Funding Opportunities	Centers for Disease Control and Prevention (CDC)
	Examples of goals:[a] 1) Number of new non-hospital focused maternal safety bundles developed; 2) number of process and outcome data measures created for new and existing non-hospital focused maternal safety bundles; and 3) number of maternal safety bundles fully integrated with contents of the peripartum racial/ethnic disparity bundle
Healthy Start Initiative supplemental funding	*Funding details:* In 2019, HRSA awarded about $12 million in supplemental funding (about $140,000 per year) to 85 award recipients in addition to base funding that these recipients received for the primary purpose of the Healthy Start Program.[b] *Purpose*: Provides support for recipients to hire clinical providers to provide direct access to well-woman care as well as maternity care aimed at reducing adverse pregnancy outcomes among high-risk and underserved women. These clinical providers will also support health educators by conducting training on the identification of maternal early warning signs in order to prevent obstetric emergencies often related to maternal mortality and severe maternal morbidity. *Examples of goals:*[a] 1)The percent of programs promoting and/or facilitating timely prenatal care; 2) the percent of programs promoting and/or facilitating timely postpartum care; and 3) the percent of programs promoting and/or facilitating well-woman visits/preventive health care.
Rural Maternity and Obstetrics Management Strategies Program	*Funding details*: In 2019, HRSA awarded 3 4-year cooperative agreements to Bexar County Hospital District in San Antonio, Texas, Saint Francis Medical Center in Cape Girardeau, Missouri, and Taos Health Systems, Inc. in Taos, New Mexico with up to $600,000 in funding the first year for a total funding amount of about $1.8 million across all awardees. Future funding amounts are contingent upon availability. *Purpose:* Supports efforts to improve access to and continuity of maternal and obstetrics care in rural communities. *Examples of goals:*[a] 1) A safe delivery environment with the support and access to specialty care for perinatal women and infants in rural communities; 2) models of maternal and obstetrics care reinforced and sustained by a payment/reimbursement structure; and 3) improved clinical outcomes for maternal and neonatal health spanning the preconception, pregnancy, labor, and delivery, and postpartum periods.

Ongoing HHS Funding Opportunities	**Centers for Disease Control and Prevention (CDC)**
State Maternal Health Innovation Program	*Funding details*: In fiscal year 2019, HRSA awarded 9 5-year cooperative agreements to Arizona, Iowa, Illinois, Maryland, Montana, North Carolina, New Jersey, Ohio and Oklahoma with up to about $2 million in annual funding for a total funding amount of about $18.7 million across all awardees. *Purpose:* Strengthens partnerships and collaboration by establishing a state-focused Maternal Health Task Force, improving state-level data surveillance on maternal mortality and severe maternal morbidity, and promoting and executing innovation in maternal health service delivery. *Examples of goals:*[a] 1) Increases within the state for the percentage of women covered by health insurance and the percentage of women who receive an annual well-woman visit; and 2) decreases within the state for the rate of pregnancy-related deaths and the racial, ethnic, and/or geographic disparities in pregnancy-related mortality rates.
Supported research	*Funding details*: HRSA supports research, including by funding it through various grants and cooperative agreements. *Purpose:* The Maternal and Child Health Bureau supports the Maternal and Child Health Extramural Research Program which provides leadership and funding for field-based, applied and translational research to advance the field of maternal and child health, improve the health and well-being of women, children, and families, and address the needs of economically or medically vulnerable maternal and child health populations.
Supported research	Within the Maternal and Child Health Bureau, the Pregnancy-Related Care Research Network assesses the clinical care patterns and educational needs of health care providers in order to support efforts to improve health care for mothers and their children, as well as for pregnant and post- partum women. *Examples of research*: Ensuring Access to High-Quality Maternity Care in Rural America, Factors Associated with High-Risk Rural Women Giving Birth in Non-NICU Hospital Settings, and Identifying Maternal Deaths in Texas Using an Enhanced Method. (See appendix IV for additional information about supported research.)
National Institutes of Health (NIH)	

Table 5. (Continued)

Ongoing HHS Funding Opportunities	Centers for Disease Control and Prevention (CDC)
Supported research	*Funding details*: NIH supports research, including by funding it through various grants, contracts, and other funding mechanisms. *Purpose:* NIH funds maternal health research through a number of its institutes and centers, such as the Eunice Kennedy Shriver National Institute of Child Health and Human Development; the National Heart, Lung, and Blood Institute, and the Office of Research on Women's Health. For example, NIH officials noted that the Eunice Kennedy Shriver National Institute of Child Health and Human Development supports essential research designed to overcome many of the complex challenges that women encounter in trying to achieve and maintain healthy pregnancies, and to prevent maternal mortality and severe maternal morbidity. *Examples of research*: Blood Pressure Trajectory and Category and Risk of Hypertensive Disorders of Pregnancy in Nulliparous Women, Recent Increases in the U.S. Maternal Mortality Rate: Disentangling Trends from Measurement Issues, Making Vital Statistics Count: Preventing U.S. Maternal Deaths Requires Better Data. (See appendix IV for additional information about supported research.)

Source: GAO analysis of HHS documents and interviews with HHS officials. | GAO-20-248.

Notes: In general, federal agencies use grants and cooperative agreements to transfer a thing of value to the recipient entity to carry out a public purpose as authorized by federal law. Cooperative agreements are used when substantial involvement by the federal agency is expected in carrying out the activity, and grants are used when substantial involvement by the federal agency is not expected. In general, federal agencies use contracts as legal instruments for the acquisition of property or services for the direct benefit or use of the federal government. See 31 U.S.C. §§ 6303-6305.

[a]Goals include outcomes, objectives, or performance measures for each funding arrangement.

[b]The Healthy Start Initiative base funding is not included because HRSA officials said the primary focus is infant mortality.

APPENDIX IV: HEALTH RESOURCES AND SERVICES ADMINISTRATION AND NATIONAL INSTITUTES OF HEALTH RESEARCH

Health Resources and Services Administration (HRSA) and National Institutes of Health (NIH) officials noted research the agencies support, including funding related to maternal health that also includes projects specific to maternal mortality or that can affect maternal mortality.

HRSA

The Maternal and Child Health Bureau supports field-based, applied and translational research through an extramural research program that provides leadership and funding that support innovative research to inform practitioners, the scientific community, and the public. According to HRSA officials, this research program helps to advance the field of maternal and child health; improve the health and well-being of women, children, and families; and address the needs of economically or medically vulnerable maternal and child health populations.

According to HRSA officials, in fiscal year 2018, HRSA awarded a total of about $1.2 million in funding for six research projects related to maternal illness. The following HRSA website includes an option for searching for funded projects using key terms, https://mchb.hrsa.gov/research/.

The following are examples of publications based on research funded by HRSA:

Surveillance of Maternal Mortality

- Baeva, S., D.L. Saxton, K. Ruggiero, et al. "Identifying Maternal Deaths in Texas Using an Enhanced Method, 2012", *Obstetrics & Gynecology*, vol. 131, no. 5 (2018): 762-769.

Maternal Health

- Casey, M.M., P. Hung, C. Henning-Smith, et al. "Rural Implications of Expanded Birth Volume Threshold for Reporting Perinatal Care Measures." *Joint Commission Journal on Quality and Patient Safety*, vol. 42, no. 4 (2016): 179-187.
- Hung, P., K.B. Kozhimannil, M.M. Casey, et al. "Why Are Obstetric Units in Rural Hospitals Closing Their Doors?" *Health Services Research*, vol. 51, no. 4 (2016): 1546-1560.
- Kozhimannil, K.B., C. Henning-Smith, P. Hung, et al. "Ensuring Access to High-Quality Maternity Care in Rural America." *Women's Health Issues*, vol. 26, no. 3 (2016): 247-250.
- Kozhimannil, K.B., P. Hung, M.M. Casey, et al. "Factors Associated with High-Risk Rural Women Giving Birth in Non-NICU Hospital Settings." *Journal of Perinatology*, vol. 36, no. 7 (2016): 510-515.
- Kozhimannil, K.B., M.M. Casey, P. Hung, et al. "Location of Childbirth for Rural Women: Implications for Maternal Levels of Care." *American Journal of Obstetrics and Gynecology*, vol. 214, no. 5 (2016): 661e1- 10.
- Kozhimannil, K.B., C. Henning-Smith, and P. Hung. "The Practice of Midwifery in Rural US Hospitals." *Journal of Midwifery & Women's Health*, vol. 61, no. 4 (2016): 411-418.
- Kozhimannil, K.B., P. Hung, M.M. Casey, et al. "Relationship between Hospital Policies for Labor Induction and Cesarean Delivery and Perinatal Care Quality among Rural U.S. Hospitals." *Journal of Health Care for the Poor and Underserved*, vol. 27, no. 4 (2016): 128-143.

- Weigel, P.A., F. Ullrich, D.M. Shane, et al. "Variation in Primary Care Service Patterns by Rural-Urban Location." *Journal of Rural Health*, vol. 32, no. 2 (2016): 196-203.

NIH

NIH support research, including funding maternal health research through a number of its institutes and centers, such as the Eunice Kennedy Shriver National Institute of Child Health and Human Development; the National Heart, Lung, and Blood Institute; the National Institute of Alcohol Abuse and Alcoholism; the National Institute of Diabetes and Digestive and Kidney Diseases; the National Institute of Mental Health; the National Institute of Nursing Research, and the Office of Research on Women's Health. For example, NIH officials noted that The *Eunice Kennedy Shriver* National Institute of Child Health and Human Development supports essential research designed to overcome many of the complex challenges that women encounter in trying to achieve and maintain healthy pregnancies, and to prevent maternal mortality and severe maternal morbidity.

In fiscal year 2018, NIH funded 661 projects totaling almost $303 million that included a focus on maternal health. The following NIH website includes a link to funded research for fiscal years 2015 through 2018 and estimates for fiscal year 2019 and 2020 by category, including maternal health, https://report.nih.gov/categorical_spending.aspx.

The following are examples of publications based on research funded by NIH:

Surveillance of Maternal Mortality

- MacDorman, M.F., E. Declercq, and M.E. Thoma. "Making Vital Statistics Count: Preventing U.S. Maternal Deaths Requires Better Data." *Obstetrics & Gynecology*, vol. 131, no. 5 (2018): 759-761.

- MacDorman, M.F., E. Declercq, H. Cabral, et al. "Recent Increases in the U.S. Maternal Mortality Rate: Disentangling Trends from Measurement Issues." *Obstetrics & Gynecology*, vol. 128, no. 3 (2016): 447-455.
- Thoma, M.E., D.A. De Silva, and M.F. MacDorman. "Examining Interpregnancy Intervals and Maternal and Perinatal Health Outcomes Using U.S. Vital Records: Important Considerations for Analysis and Interpretation." *Paediatric and Perinatal Epidemiology*, vol. 33, no. 1 (2019): O60-O72.

Maternal Health

- Brogly, S.B., K.E. Saia, M.M. Werler, et al. "Prenatal Treatment and Outcomes of Women with Opioid Use Disorder." *Obstetrics & Gynecology*, vol. 132, no. 4 (2018): 916-922.
- Dimidjian, S., S.H. Goodman, J.N. Felder, et al. "Staying Well During Pregnancy and the Postpartum: A Pilot Randomized Trial of Mindfulness-based Cognitive Therapy for the Prevention of Depressive Relapse/Recurrence." *Journal of Consulting and Clinical Psychology*, vol. 84, no. 2 (2016): 134-145.
- Hauspurg, A., S. Parry, B.M. Mercer, et al. "Blood Pressure Trajectory and Category and Risk of Hypertensive Disorders of Pregnancy in Nulliparous Women." *American Journal of Obstetrics and Gynecology*, vol. 221, no. 3 (2019): 277.e1-277.e8.
- Liu, T., M. Zhang, E. Guallar, et al. "Trace Minerals, Heavy Metals, and Preeclampsia: Findings from the Boston Birth Cohort." *Journal of the American Heart Association*, vol. 8, no. 16 (2019): e012346.

- Miller, E.C., M. Gallo, E.R. Kulick, et al. "Infections and Risk of Peripartum Stroke during Delivery Admissions." *Stroke*, vol. 49, no. 5 (2018): 1129-1134.
- Sheen, J.J., J. D. Wright, D. Goffman, et al. "Maternal Age and Risk for Adverse Outcomes." *American Journal of Obstetrics and Gynecology*, vol. 219, no. 4 (2018): 390.e1-390.e15.

APPENDIX V: MATERNAL MORTALITY EFFORTS IN SELECTED STATES

To describe how selected states use Department of Health and Human Services (HHS) funds to implement select efforts to reduce maternal mortality, we interviewed officials from five states—California, Georgia, Illinois, Maryland, and Texas—selected because of their geographic diversity and because these state have the following efforts shown in Table 6. Officials from three of the five states we interviewed said that the Alliance for Innovation on Maternal Health (AIM) Initiative had an immediate or the largest effect on addressing maternal mortality in their state. Officials from the other two states said they could not identify which efforts had the largest or most immediate effect on addressing maternal mortality. Officials from one state noted the importance of a collaborative approach and the other noted that there is no one contributing factor for maternal mortality. Some of the HHS-funded efforts previously described in appendix III had not been awarded at the time of our interviews, such as the State Maternal Health Innovation Program cooperative agreements. See Table 6 below for information about these states' efforts.

Table 6. Selected State Efforts to Reduce Maternal Mortality

California	
Maternal and Child Health (MCH) Services Block Grant	• Recipient: The California Department of Public Health, Maternal, Child and Adolescent Health Division is the recipient of the MCH Services Block Grant. • Federal and overall expenditures: California's fiscal year 2017 MCH Services Block Grant expenditures totaled over \$3.8 billion, almost \$42 million of which were federal expenditures. Over \$37 million of the total spending was for pregnant women.[a] • Women and maternal health priorities: The 2017 priority need for women and maternal health was to improve access and utilization to comprehensive, quality health services for women. • National Performance Measure and National Outcome Measure: With regard to women and maternal health, California tracks progress against the following National Performance Measure— percent of women ages 18-44 with a preventive visit in the past year, which is related to the maternal mortality National Outcome Measure—maternal mortality rate per 100,000 live births. • Other points of interest: MCH Services Block Grant funds support the Black Infant Health Program, which officials said helps address maternal morbidity and mortality of black mothers in the late maternal period.
Maternal Mortality Review Committee (MMRC)	• Date established: California's Pregnancy Associated Mortality Review was established in 2006 after a concerning increase in maternal mortality. • Latest report: According to officials, their latest MMRC report, as of September 2019, that covers pregnancy-related deaths from obstetric and other medical causes was published in 2018 for deaths that occurred from 2002 through 2007. In 2019, the MMRC published a special report that covers pregnancy-associated suicides that occurred from 2002 through 2012. • Federal funding: (1) Officials said California uses the MCH Services Block Grant to fund staff time and resources for the MMRC. (2) According to Centers for Disease Control and Prevention (CDC) officials, in 2019, California was awarded a cooperative agreement with CDC.[b] • Use of MMRIA: As of May 2019, officials said the MMRC was not submitting the results of their reviews to CDC using Maternal Mortality Review Information Application (MMRIA)—an electronic application for collecting and sharing MMRC results. The MMRC will be expected to use MMRIA in accordance with the 2019 cooperative agreement with CDC that requires recipients to share this information within 2 years of a death.

California	
	• Other points of interest: According to officials, California recently implemented a rapid case review model, where committee members discuss cases through electronic communication. In this model, committee members only identify the cause of death and relationship to pregnancy. Quality improvement opportunities and preventability are not assessed in the rapid case review model. Officials said this will improve the timeliness and accuracy of their data on maternal deaths up to 1 year after the end of pregnancy
Perinatal Quality Collaborative (PQC) and Alliance for Innovation on Maternal Health (AIM)	• Date established: California's Maternal Quality Care Collaborative was established in 2006 and uses research, quality improvement toolkits, state-wide outreach collaboratives and a Maternal Data Center to improve health outcomes for mothers and infants. • Federal funding: According to CDC officials, California's collaborative received funding through cooperative agreements awarded by CDC in 2011 and 2014. • AIM bundle implementation: According to officials, California's Maternal Quality Care Collaborative works closely with AIM in the development of the maternal safety bundles and then develops toolkits that provide evidence-based guidance for implementing best practices to improve clinical care in obstetrics. • Use of data center: According to officials, California's collaborative used its 2011 PQC grant funding from CDC to develop the California Maternal Data Center. They also said that the Maternal Data Center allows hospitals to view their quality of care in real time and compare themselves to similar hospitals. Birth outcome measures tracked in the data center are broken out by racial group so California can work to address the disparities in birth outcomes. • Other points of interest: California officials cited continued concern about racial disparities in maternal mortality in their states. As such, officials stated the collaborative is developing a Birth Equity Collaborative to improve birth care, experiences and outcomes for, by and with Black mothers and birthing people in California.
Georgia	
Maternal and Child Health (MCH) Services Block Grant	• Recipient: The Georgia Department of Public Health is the recipient of the MCH Services Block Grant. • Federal and overall expenditures: Georgia's fiscal year 2017 MCH Services Block grant expenditures totaled about $283 million, almost $17 million of which were federal expenditures. Over $23 million of total spending was for pregnant women.[a] • Women and maternal health priorities: The 2017 priority need for women and maternal health was to prevent maternal mortality.

Table 6. (Continued)

Georgia	
Maternal and Child Health (MCH) Services Block Grant	• National Performance Measure and National Outcome Measure: With regard to women and maternal health, Georgia tracks progress against the following National Performance Measure— percent of women, ages 18 through 44, with a preventive medical visit in the past year, which is related to the maternal mortality National Outcome Measure—maternal mortality rate per 100,000 live births. • Other points of interest: Officials said they have ideas for future project using their MCH Services Block Grant funds that include grants to community partners working to address specific causes of maternal mortality.
Maternal Mortality Review Committee (MMRC)	• Date established: According to officials, Georgia's MMRC was re-established in 2013 after a period of inactivity, when physicians and state officials became aware of an increase in maternal deaths. • Latest report: According to officials, their latest MMRC report, as of September 2019, was issued in 2019 and covers deaths that occurred in 2014 as well as aggregate data for 2012-2014. • Federal funding: Officials said the MCH Services Block Grant is the primary source of funding for the MMRC. • Use of MMRIA: According to officials, Georgia began submitting case abstraction and MMRC case review findings into MMRIA in April 2017.The MMRC has shared results of their reviews for inclusion in two multi-state publications issued in 2018 and 2019. • Other points of interest: Officials said the Department of Public Heath leads the Georgia PQC that serves as the action arm of the MMRC. The Georgia PQC utilizes findings and recommendations from the MMRC to implement maternal quality improvement initiatives.
Perinatal Quality Collaborative (PQC) and Alliance for Innovation on Maternal Health (AIM)	• Date established: Georgia's PQC was established in 2012 to identify and implement quality improvement strategies to improve maternal and neonatal care and outcomes. • Federal funding: (1) According to CDC officials, in 2017, Georgia's PQC was awarded a 3-year cooperative agreement with CDC. (2) According to state officials, the PQC will be eligible to receive $9,000 annually from AIM to support implementation of AIM maternal safety bundles.

Illinois	
	• AIM bundle implementation: In 2018, Georgia's PQC implemented the Obstetric Hemorrhage AIM bundle based on the MMRC's finding that hemorrhage was a leading cause of death in Georgia. Forty-four of the state's hospitals were implementing this bundle as of March 2019. • Use of a data center: According to officials, Georgia's Department of Public Health submits structure and process measure data to the AIM Data Center for each participating hospital. DPH utilizes hospital discharge data to monitor the impact of quality improvement initiatives on maternal outcomes. • Other points of interest: Officials said the PQC has a Health Equities Subcommittee that is exploring opportunities to address racial/ethnic disparities in maternal and neonatal health in the state
Maternal and Child Health (MCH) Services Block Grant	• Recipient: The Illinois Department of Public Health is the recipient of the MCH Services Block Grant. • Federal and overall expenditures: Illinois's fiscal year 2017 MCH Services Block Grant expenditures totaled over $52 million, almost $21 million of which were federal expenditures. Almost $12 million of the total spending was for pregnant women.[a] • Women and maternal health priorities: The 2017 priority need for women and maternal health was to assure accessibility, availability and quality of preventive and primary care for all women, particularly for women of reproductive age. • National Performance Measure and National Outcome Measure: With regard to women and maternal health, Illinois tracks progress against the following National Performance Measure— percent of women, ages 18 through 44, with preventive medical visit in the past year, which is related to the maternal mortality National Outcome Measure—maternal mortality rate per 100,000 live births. • Other points of interest: Officials said they are planning to address disparities through a multiyear approach that includes identifying barriers to care for minority and at risk populations and eventually using MCH Services Block grant funds to support community organizations to overcome these barriers.
Maternal Mortality Review Committee (MMRC)	• Date established: Illinois' MMRC was established in 2000. • Latest report: According to officials, the latest MMRC report, as of September 2019, was published in 2018 and covers deaths that occurred in 2015. • Federal funding: (1) Officials said the MCH Services Block Grant funds the MMRC. (2) According to CDC officials, in 2019, Illinois was awarded a cooperative agreement with CDC.[b]

Table 6. (Continued)

Illinois	
Maternal Mortality Review Committee (MMRC)	• Use of MMRIA: Officials said the MMRC began submitting the results of their reviews to CDC's MMRIA in March 2019, after working with CDC on implementation. The MMRC will be expected to continue using MMRIA in accordance with the 2019 cooperative agreement with CDC that requires recipients to share this information within 2 years of a death. • Other points of interest: Illinois has two MMRCs. The second MMRC, established in 2015, is focused on violent deaths—homicide, suicide, and drug overdose.
Perinatal Quality Collaborative (PQC) and Alliance for Innovation on Maternal Health (AIM)	• Date established: Illinois's PQC was established in 2012 to use data-driven, evidence-based practices and improves perinatal quality resulting in improved birth outcomes, improved health for women and infants, and decreased costs in Illinois. • Federal funding: According to CDC officials, in 2014 and 2017, Illinois's PQC was awarded a 3-year cooperative agreement from CDC. • AIM bundle implementation: According to officials, in 2016 Illinois's PQC began implementing the Severe Hypertension in Pregnancy AIM maternal safety bundle. Additionally, in 2018 the PQC implemented the Obstetric Care for Women with Opioid Use Disorder AIM bundle. As of May 2019, 119 hospitals were participating in at least one PQC initiative. • Use of a data center: According to officials, Illinois's PQC used early funding from the Children's Health Insurance Program Reauthorization Act of 2009 to develop a rapid-response data system and CDC funding supports the data system ongoing development. The hospitals use Illinois's PQC data system and not the AIM data system to implement quality improvement initiatives, and Illinois's PQC submits de-identified data to AIM. • Other points of interest: Officials said they are working to develop a birth equity initiative to address racial disparities in the state to launch in 2021.
Maryland	
Maternal and Child Health (MCH) Services Block Grant	• Recipient: The Maryland Department of Health is the recipient of the MCH Services Block Grant. • Federal and overall expenditures: Maryland's fiscal year 2017 MCH Services Block Grant expenditures totaled about $20 million, almost $12 million of which were federal expenditures. Over $2 million of the total spending was for pregnant women.[a].

Maryland	
	• Women and maternal health priorities: The 2017 priority needs for women and maternal health were to optimize the health and well-being of girls and women across the life span using preventive strategies and to reduce substance use/abuse across the life span for MCH populations including use of tobacco products, alcohol, prescription drugs and opioids. • National Performance Measure and National Outcome Measure: With regard to women and maternal health, Maryland tracks progress against the following National Performance Measure— percent of cesarean deliveries among low-risk first births and percent of women who smoke during pregnancy, which are related to the maternal mortality National Outcome Measure—maternal mortality rate per 100,000 live births. • Other points of interest: Officials said they used the MCH Services Block Grant to establish an effort called Babies Born Healthy Program—originally designed to address infant mortality—which has been expanded to provide care coordination to mothers from three months to 1 year post pregnancy as a way to address the disparities in the state's maternal mortality
Maternal Mortality Review Committee (MMRC)	• Date established: Maryland's Maternal Mortality Review Program, which includes an MMRC, was established by in 2000. • Latest report: According to officials, the latest MMRC report, as of September 2019, was published in 2018 and covers deaths that occurred in 2016. The MMRC has published annual reports since 2002. • Federal funding: According to officials, Maryland uses the MCH Services Block Grant to fund a contract with the state's medical society to prepare cases for the MMRC to review. • Use of MMRIA: As of June 2019, officials said the MMRC was not submitting the results of its review to CDC using MMRIA, but plan to begin using MMRIA in 2020 for their review of deaths that occurred in 2018. • Other points of interest: Officials said that the Maryland state legislature established a stakeholder group—advocacy and community group representatives—to and community group representatives— to help facilitate looking at the MMRC's findings through a lens of disparity.

Table 6. (Continued)

Maryland	
Perinatal Quality Collaborative (PQC) and Alliance for Innovation on Maternal Health (AIM)	• Date established: The Maryland Patient Safety Center started Maryland's PQC in 2007 to improve maternal and infant health and to reduce severe maternal and infant morbidity and mortality through education, collaboration and implementation of evidence-based interventions. • Federal funding: According to officials, the PQC receives a small funding award of $9,000 annually through AIM to support implementation of AIM maternal safety bundles.
	• AIM bundle implementation: Officials said Maryland's PQC implemented the Safe Reduction of Primary Cesarean Section Birth AIM bundle, which ended in 2018. The PQC continues to monitor the hospitals' sustainability of the bundle. In 2019, the PQC implemented the Obstetric Care for Women with Opioid Use Disorder AIM bundle. • Use of data center: Officials said they use and automated process for inputting data into the AIM Data Center. • Other points of interest: According to officials, the PQC is considering programming to address racial disparities in maternal mortality, including the possible addition of unconscious bias courses to its patient safety education programs.
Texas	
Maternal and Child Health (MCH) Services Block Grant	• Recipient: The Texas Department of State Health Services is the recipient of the MCH Services Block Grant. • Federal and overall expenditures: Texas's fiscal year 2017 MCH Services Block Grant expenditures totaled over $72 million, almost $34 million of which were federal expenditures. Almost $11 million of the total spending was for pregnant women.[a] • Women and maternal health priorities: The 2017 priority need for women and maternal health was to ensure use of culturally and linguistically appropriate Maternal and Child Health education and outreach efforts. • National Performance Measure (NPM) and National Outcome Measure (NOM): With regard to women and maternal health, Texas tracks progress against the following National Performance Measure—percent of women who smoke during pregnancy, which is related to the maternal mortality National Outcome Measure—maternal mortality rate per 100,000 live births.

Texas	
	• Other points of interest: Officials said their MCH Services Block Grant funds programs that address health disparities, including the Texas Healthy Mothers and Babies Coalition that provides funding for staff to specific community groups working to remove barriers to care for people in their community.
Maternal Mortality Review Committee (MMRC)	• Date established: Texas's Maternal Mortality and Morbidity Task Force was established in 2013. The name was changed to the Texas Maternal Mortality and Morbidity Review Committee. • Latest report: According to officials, the MMRC's latest report, as of September 2019, was published in 2018 and covers deaths that occurred in 2012. Officials noted the report also included analyses of 2012 through 2015 data and a summary of a Department of State Health Services study published 2018, which used an enhanced method to calculate a more accurate maternal mortality rate for Texas in 2012. • Federal funding: (1) According to officials their MMRC has been exclusively funded by the MCH Services Block Grant. (2) According to CDC officials, in 2019, Texas was awarded a cooperative agreement with CDC.[b] • Use of MMRIA: As of May 2019, officials said the MMRC was not submitting the results of their review to CDC using MMRIA, but officials said they were working with CDC to address challenges to its implementation. The MMRC will be expected to use MMRIA in accordance with the 2019 cooperative agreement with CDC that requires recipients to share this information within 2 years of a death. • Other points of interest: Officials said Texas's committee meetings are public and media, legislators, and others have participated.

Table 6. (Continued)

Texas	
Perinatal Quality Collaborative (PQC) and Alliance for Innovation on Maternal Health (AIM)	• Date established: Texas's Collaborative for Healthy Mothers and Babies began operating in 2013 to advance health care quality and patient safety for all Texas mothers and babies. According to officials, in 2017, Texas also established TexasAIM in collaboration with the hospital association to guide the implementation of maternal safety bundles. • Federal funding: Officials said the MCH Services Block Grant provides funding for Texas's Collaborative for Healthy Mothers and Babies and funding for TexasAIM's implementation of AIM maternal safety bundles. • AIM bundle implementation: According to officials, TexasAIM began implementing the Obstetric Hemorrhage AIM bundle in 2018. In 2021, they will implement the Obstetric Care for Women with Opioid Use Disorder AIM bundle. • Use of data center: Officials said that Texas Department of State Health Services staff submit outcome measures and hospital staff submit quarterly structure and process measures into the AIM Data Center. • Other points of interest: According to officials, Texas's Collaborative for Healthy Mothers and Babies used AIM's information on Maternal Early Warning Signs, which provides the steps necessary to identify risk early.

Source: GAO analysis of Department of Health and Human Services (HHS) and state documents and interviews with HHS and state officials. | GAO-20-248.

Note: unless otherwise specified, the use of officials refers to state officials.

[a]Data for FY 2017 expenditures were the latest available as of October 2019.

[b]In 2019, CDC awarded 5-year Supporting Maternal Mortality Review Committee cooperative agreements. These agreements support a MMRC's ability to collect the most detailed, complete data on causes and circumstances surrounding pregnancy-related deaths to develop recommendations for prevention. This multidisciplinary approach encourages collaboration with clinical and non-clinical partnerships to improve quality of care and address social determinants of health to reduce health inequities.

In: Maternal Mortality
Editor: Mathias T. Gregersen
ISBN: 978-1-53618-161-6

Chapter 2

BETTER DATA AND BETTER OUTCOMES: REDUCING MATERNAL MORTALITY IN THE U.S.*

Subcommittee on Health

Thursday, September 27, 2018
House of Representatives, Committee on Energy and Commerce,
Washington, DC.

The subcommittee met, pursuant to call, at 10:00 a.m., in room 2123 Rayburn House Office Building, Hon. Michael Burgess (chairman of the subcommittee) presiding.

Members present: Representatives Burgess, Guthrie, Barton, Shimkus, Latta, Lance, Griffith, Bilirakis, Long, Bucshon, Brooks, Mullin, Hudson, Carter, Walden(ex officio), Green, Engel, Schakowsky, Castor, Schrader, Kennedy, Ca´rdenas, DeGette, and Pallone (ex officio).

---

* This is an edited, reformatted and augmented version of Hearing before the Subcommittee on Health, of the Committee on Energy and Commerce, House of Representatives, One Hundred Fifteenth Congress, Second Session, Serial No. 115–169, dated September 27, 2018.

Staff present: Mike Bloomquist, Staff Director; Samantha Bopp, Staff Assistant; Daniel Butler, Staff Assistant; Adam Fromm, Director of Outreach and Coalitions; Zach Hunter, Director of Communications; Ed Kim, Policy Coordinator, Health; Ryan Long, Deputy Staff Director; Drew McDowell, Executive Assistant; Brannon Rains, Staff Assistant; Austin Stonebraker, Press Assistant; Josh Trent, Deputy Chief Health Counsel, Health; Hamlin Wade, Special Advisor, External Affairs; Jacquelyn Bolen, Minority Professional Staff; Jeff Carroll, Minority Staff Director; Evan Gilbert, Minority Press Assistant; Waverly Gordon, Minority Health Counsel; Tiffany Guarascio, Minority Deputy Staff Director and Chief Health Advisor; Tim Robinson, Minority Chief Counsel; and Samantha Satchell, Minority Policy Analyst.

OPENING STATEMENT OF HON. MICHAEL C. BURGESS, A REPRESENTATIVE IN CONGRESS FROM THE STATE OF TEXAS

Mr. BURGESS. And the Subcommittee on Health will now come to order. I recognize myself 5 minutes for purpose of an opening statement. And I want to thank everyone for joining us this morning to discuss a topic that is important to each and every one of us. This is a subject matter that has been brought to the forefront by members of this subcommittee, members of Congress generally, actions of state legislators, and the media.

Having spent 3 decades myself practicing OB/GYN, I believe it should be a national goal to eliminate all preventable maternal mortality. Even a single maternal death is too many. All too often we have read about the stories of seemingly healthy pregnant women who are thrilled to be having a child and then to everyone's surprise suffers severe complications, death, or near death during a pregnancy, birth, or postpartum. The death of a new or expecting mother is a tragic event that devastates everyone involved, and if there are preventable scenarios we need to do what we can to stop that.

The alarming trend in our country's rate of maternal mortality first came to my attention in September 2016 reading a copy of the American College of Obstetricians and Gynecologists, The Green Journal. The original research found that the maternal mortality rate had increased in 48 states and Washington, D.C. from 2000 to 2014, while the international trend was moving in the opposite direction. Since reading that article, I have spoken to providers, hospital administrators, state task forces, and public health experts. The more I looked into this troubling issue, the more I realized that we have got much more we need to understand.

This subcommittee had an informational briefing last year on this topic to inform members and to start the road toward this hearing. This is an issue that we cannot solve without accurate data. There were efforts in our nation to address maternal and infant mortality in the first half of the 20th century and the data showed that these efforts were indeed successful.

But according to the Centers for Disease Control and Prevention the United States' maternal mortality rate, 7.2 deaths per 100,000 in 1999 and increased to 18 deaths per 100,000 live births in 2014. The Centers for Disease Control began conducting national surveillance of pregnancy related deaths in 1986 due to a lack of data on causes of maternal death.

In 2003, the Centers for Disease Control National Center for Health Statistics revised standards for certain death certificates and added a pregnancy checkbox. While this checkbox has led to increased data collection on maternal deaths, it does not provide enough insight as to why or how these deaths occurred. Representative Jaime Herrera Beutler joining us this morning, the discussion draft that she has put forward will address the complex issue of maternal mortality by enabling states to form maternal mortality review committees to evaluate, improve, and standardize their maternal death rate.

This is a critical step in the right direction as physicians, public health officials, and Congress are unable to reach conclusions based upon current data as to what the causes for maternal mortality increases are. Once we establish what these are, there will be an opportunity to use the data to implement the best practices toward a solution.

Texas is a good example of a state that has enacted legislation to create and sustain a Maternal Mortality and Morbidity Task Force. Texas has put time and effort in funding and to reviewing maternal deaths in order to find the trends in the increases and the causes of death. The Task Force's September 2018 report, which I have here and later on we will ask unanimous consent to be made part of the record, stated that the leading causes of pregnancy-related death in 2012 included cardiovascular, obstetric hemorrhage, infection sepsis, and cardiomyopathy.

This chapter is just a snapshot of the national picture as causes do vary from state to state. Additionally, this May, various researchers involved in the review of Texas' maternal deaths published a paper, again in The Green Journal, detailing that unintentional user error and other issues led to inaccurate reporting of maternal mortality. The researchers concluded that relying solely on obstetric codes for identifying maternal deaths appears to be insufficient and can lead to inaccurate ratios.

The moral of this story is we must ensure accurate data to accurately pinpoint the clinical issues contributing to these tragic deaths. I would like to submit a statement for the record from Dr. Gary Hankins and, without objection, so ordered, the chairman of the Department of OB/GYN at the University of Texas Medical Branch in Galveston.

[The information appears at the conclusion of the hearing.]

Mr. BURGESS. And Dr. Hankins was one of those doctors who briefed us during the briefing last year. Dr. Hankins has subspecialty training in maternal fetal medicine and served as vice chair for the Texas Morbidity and Mortality Review Committee.

At one time we were scheduled to be joined by Dr. Lisa Hollier, also of Texas, who is also part of that committee. I think we had to postpone last week because of a hurricane and she could not accommodate the reschedule. But Dr. Hollier has also been integral in working on this at the state level.

So I certainly look forward to hearing from our panel of witnesses today as how we can address this vital and devastating issue.

[The prepared statement of Mr. Burgess follows:]

PREPARED STATEMENT OF HON. MICHAEL C. BURGESS

Good morning. Thank you to everyone for joining us this morning to discuss a topic that is important to each and every one of us, maternal mortality. This is a subject matter that has been brought to the forefront by Members of this Subcommittee, actions of State Legislatures, and the media. Having spent nearly three decades as an OB/GYN, I believe it should be a national goal to eliminate all preventable maternal mortality—even a single maternal death is too many.

All too often do we read about stories of seemingly healthy pregnant women who are thrilled to be having a child, and to everyone's surprise, suffers severe complications, or death during pregnancy, birth, or post-partum. The death of a new or expecting mother is a tragic event that devastates everyone involved, but in many cases these are preventable scenarios.

The alarming trend in our country's rate of maternal mortality first came to my attention in September 2016, when I was reading my copy of the Green Journal. The original research found that the maternal mortality rate increased in 48 states and Washington DC from 2000 to 2014, while the international trend was moving in the opposite direction. Since reading that article, I have spoken with providers, hospital administrators, state task forces, and public health experts. The more I dove into this troubling issue, the more I realized how little we understand. This Subcommittee held an informational briefing last year on this topic to inform members and pave the road to this hearing.

This is an issue that we cannot solve without accurate data. There were great efforts in our nation to address maternal and infant mortality in the first half of the 20th Century, and the data showed that those efforts were successful. Yet, according to the Centers for Disease Control and Prevention (CDC), the U.S. maternal mortality rate was 7.2 deaths per 100,000 live births in 1999, and increased to 18 deaths per 100,000 live births in 2014.

CDC began conducting national surveillance of pregnancy-related deaths in 1986 due to a lack of data on causes of maternal death. In 2003, the CDC National Center for Health Statistics revised standards for certain death certificates, and added a pregnancy checkbox. While this checkbox has led to increased data collection on maternal deaths, it does not provide enough insight into why or how these mothers are dying.

Representative Jamie Herrera-Beutler's discussion draft will address the complex issue of maternal mortality by enabling States to form maternal mortality review committees to evaluate, improve, and standardize their maternal death data. This is a critical step in the right direction, as physicians, public health officials, and Congress are unable to reach conclusions based upon current data as to what the causes for maternal mortality are. Once we establish what these are, there will be an opportunity to use the data to implement best practices.

Texas is a great example of a state that has enacted legislation to create and sustain a maternal mortality and morbidity task force. Texas has put much time, effort, and funding into reviewing maternal deaths in order to find trends in the causes of death. The Task Force's September 2018 report stated that leading causes of pregnancy-related death in 2012 included cardiovascular and coronary conditions, obstetric hemorrhage, infection/sepsis, and cardiomyopathy. This chapter is just a snapshot of the national picture, as causes vary from state to state.

Additionally, this May, various researchers involved in the review of Texas maternal deaths published a paper in the Green Journal detailing that unintentional user error and other issues led to inaccurate reporting of maternal mortality. The researchers also concluded that "relying solely on obstetric codes for identifying maternal deaths appears to be insufficient and can lead to inaccurate maternal mortality ratios." The moral of this story is that we must ensure accurate data to accurately pinpoint the clinical issues contributing to these tragic deaths.

I would like to submit a statement for the record from Dr. Gary Hankins, Chairman of the Department of OB/GYN at The University of Texas Medical Branch. He has subspecialty training in Maternal Fetal Medicine and served as Vice Chair for the Texas Maternal Morbidity and Mortality Review Committee.

I look forward to hearing from our expert panel of witnesses as to how we can address this vital yet devastating issue.

Mr. BURGESS. The chair recognizes the ranking member of the subcommittee, Mr. Green, 5 minutes for your opening statement, please.

Opening Statement of Hon. Gene Green, a Representative in Congress from the State of Texas

Mr. GREEN. Thank you, Mr. Chairman, for calling today's hearing on maternal mortality in the United States, and I would also like to thank our colleague who is in our distinguished panelists for joining us this morning.

I would like to take just a moment, Mr. Chairman. My deputy chief of staff, LD/LA, Sergio Espinosa, this will be his last committee hearing and he has been working with me on health care in our office for many years—8 years, it has been 8 or 9. This is his last hearing. And those of you who someday decide you are not going to run for reelection, you will know that you will be losing staff members in the last 2 or 3 months. But I just want to thank Sergio for his work in the office on many issues, but particularly in the last number of months on health care.

So—and I will continue with my statement.

[Applause.]

Mr. GREEN. The Centers for Disease Control and Prevention reports that more than 700 women in the United States die each year due to complications related to pregnancy and childbirth, and more than 50,000 women experience a life-threatening complication. Maternal mortality in our country has more than doubled between 1987 and 2014, from 7.2 to 18 maternal deaths per 100,000 live births. In comparison, a recent World Health Organization study found that maternal mortality is on the decline in 157 of the 183 countries.

These numbers are troubling as we are because even more acute when you look at the existing racial, socioeconomic, and geographic disparities, for example, African American women are nearly three times as likely to die of complications relating to pregnancy and childbirth compared to white women. In America in the 21st century, no woman should ever die of complications related to pregnancy and childbirth.

Congress has a duty to act and reverse this terrible trend. I would like to thank my colleagues both Congresswoman Diane DeGette and Congresswoman Jaime Herrera Beutler for offering their discussion draft, The Preventing Maternal Deaths Act that will help protect pregnant and postpartum mothers. This legislation will provide grants to states and tribes to help establish and support already existing maternal mortality review committees, MMRCs, to identify and review pregnancy-related and pregnancy-associated deaths.

MMRCs which are currently operating in over 30 states have been helping strengthen public health surveillance by linking vital data to the multidisciplinary healthcare professionals practicing in women's health. I support the bipartisan legislation and hope our committee will recommend it in consideration before the full House before the end of the year.

My Preventing Maternal Deaths Act is an important first step. Our committee can and must do more to protect our nation's mothers. Despite the gains made under the Affordable Care Act, nearly one in seven women of childbearing age remain uninsured. The biggest barrier to women of childbearing age receiving healthcare coverage is continuing refusal of 19 states, including my home State of Texas, to expand Medicaid. Continuing of a comprehensive health insurance is critical for expecting and postpartum mothers to receive the post and postnatal care they need for themselves and their babies.

Medical research shows chronic conditions such as hypertension, diabetes, heart disease, and obesity which are becoming more common for expecting mothers can increase their risk for complications during pregnancy. Ensuring continuing of coverage preceding pregnancy will help women of childbearing age best manage these chronic conditions before they become a problem.

Last year I introduced Incentivizing Medicaid Expansion Act, H.R. 2688, in order to incentivize states to provide critical Medicaid coverage for uninsured Americans and avoid the kinds of tragedy that has led to the rising rate of mortality in my home State. My legislation would guarantee that the Federal Government covers a hundred percent of expansion costs for the first 3 years for states that have not yet expanded, and no less than 90 percent afterwards. I ask the committee to give this legislation the serious consideration that it deserves and help reverse the public health crisis that maternal mortality and severe maternal morbidity have become too many for our communities and our country.

And in my last 39 seconds, UTMB in Galveston has been the catchment for most of the births in East Texas and South Texas and for decades, and I appreciate that university and that medical school for doing that for our families. In the Houston area we have a hospital district, but Medicaid would at least help get them reimbursed. But UTMB is the catchment for problem pregnancies in South Texas and East Texas.

Thank you, Mr. Chairman. I yield back.

Mr. BURGESS. The chair thanks the gentleman. The gentleman yields back. The chair recognizes the gentleman from Oregon, the chairman of the full committee, Mr. Walden, 5 minutes for your opening statement, please.

OPENING STATEMENT OF HON. GREG WALDEN, A REPRESENTATIVE IN CONGRESS FROM THE STATE OF OREGON

Mr. WALDEN. Well, thank you, Chairman Burgess.

Doctor, we are glad that you are chairing this subcommittee and this subcommittee hearing especially given your many decades of real-world experiences in OB/GYN. So we are glad to have you at the helm for this hearing especially. It is a difficult topic and it is one that is close to many of us.

Far too many mothers die because of complications during pregnancy, and the effects of such a tragedy on any family is impossible to fully understand. What is both surprising and devastating is that despite massive innovation and advances in health care and technology we have experienced recent reports that have indicated that the number of women dying due to pregnancy complications is actually increasing. It is actually going up.

According to the Centers for Disease Control and Prevention, maternal mortality rates in America have more than doubled since 1987, and I think we are all asking how can that be? Well, this is not a statistic any of us wants to hear. There are questions as to whether the increases due to data collection are broader questions about healthcare delivery. The bill before us today will help us answer these really important questions and hopefully ensure that expectant newborn mothers receive even better care.

I want to thank Congresswoman Herrera Beutler, my neighbor to the north in Washington State, for bringing this issue to our attention. She has been a real leader on this effort for many, many months, if not years. And especially given what you have been through in your own situation, we are proud of you and of your children and so we are glad to have you before the committee.

I also want to thank my colleague and friend from Colorado, Diana DeGette, for her partnership on the draft legislation that is before us today. She has been a real leader on 21st Century Cures and other public health issues that are so important. And I want to extend a sincere thank you to the members of our second panel. Mr. Johnson, it is good to see you again. We appreciate you coming back here. I am sorry for what you have been through, but I appreciate your willingness to come share with us. Your testimony makes a difference in public policy.

The draft bill we are examining today is the Preventing Maternal Deaths Act of 2018. The bill would enhance our Federal efforts to support maternal mortality review committees in each of our states. And earlier this year, the Oregon legislature passed a bill to establish such a committee in my home State which brings a wide range of medical providers together with community organizations and with public health experts to study maternal mortality and figure out its underlying causes. That information and lessons learned will then be shared with law enforcement and healthcare providers across Oregon. Congress should support and it should build off of these efforts and others across the country so many of these deaths could be prevented if best practices for maternal health care were followed and more widely understood.

So that is what this hearing is all about. We appreciate you being here and we look forward to the testimony from our other panelists and of course from our colleague. I will tell you in advance we actually have two subcommittees going on simultaneously, and as chairman of the overall committee I have to bounce back and forth between them. But thank you for being here and we look forward to moving forward to find solutions.

And with that, Mr. Chairman, I yield back.

Mr. BURGESS. The chair thanks the gentleman. The gentleman yields back. The chair recognizes the gentleman from New Jersey, Mr. Pallone, the ranking member of the full committee, 5 minutes for an opening statement, please.

Opening Statement of Hon. Frank Pallone, Jr., a Representative in Congress from the State of New Jersey

Mr. PALLONE. Thank you, Mr. Chairman. Hundreds of women die each year from pregnancy-related or pregnancy-associated complications in the United States, and more than 60 percent of these deaths are preventable. Shamefully, the maternal mortality rate in the U.S. has increased while most of the rest of the developed world has actually fallen. And this is not just alarming, it is unconscionable. We have a responsibility to understand why this is happening and what we should be doing to combat this crisis.

Mr. Green and I wrote a letter to Chairman Burgess and Chairman Walden on this issue in May and I am pleased we are finally holding a hearing today. Today we will discuss a draft of the Preventing Maternal Deaths Act, which mirrors a version that passed out of the Senate Health

Committee. This is a good bill. It is critical that we have the necessary data to understand the underlying causes of maternal deaths and identify strategies that can help us combat it.

This bill encourages states to implement maternal mortality review committees to study this data and make recommendations on ways to combat maternal death. Review committees that are diverse and interdisciplinary can identify trends, patterns, and disparities that contribute to preventable maternal deaths. And with this information, healthcare providers can monitor the effectiveness of their policy and practice changes.

Now my home State of New Jersey was the second state in the nation to institute a maternal mortality review committee which has worked extensively to review New Jersey's maternal death cases to better understand their root causes and prevent deaths in the future. However, New Jersey's maternal mortality rate remains much too high and much more work still needs to be done.

Extensive public reporting has vividly described the risks American woman face in childbirth and the postpartum period and has also highlighted the vast disparities in outcome. While women of all backgrounds are at risk for pregnancy-related complications, it is critical we also examine why maternal death rates are disproportionately higher for women of color, low-income women, and women living in rural areas. And we must understand why, and work together to address these disparities.

However, we must also consider other ways we can combat maternal mortality, including by expanding health insurance coverage and ensuring all women have access to the reproductive health services they need. Unfortunately, efforts by the Trump administration to sabotage the Affordable Care Act, curtail the Medicaid program, and limit family planning services have only served to harm women and their families. Reducing maternal deaths in the United States must be a public health priority. I look forward to working with my colleagues to advance this bill and to begin addressing this crisis in a meaningful way.

And I would like to now yield 2 minutes to my colleague, the Democratic sponsor of H.R. 1318, Ms. DeGette.

Ms. DEGETTE. Thank you very much for yielding.

Mr. Chairman, thank you so much for having this hearing. And I know my co-sponsor, Congresswoman Herrera Beutler, and I very much hope that we can mark this bill up and pass it during the lame duck session. In my opinion, it has been far too delayed given what we are seeing in this country.

Maternal mortality rose in the United States between 2000 and 2014 by 26 percent. This is really shocking to people who I talk to about this because other developed nations in the world have slashed their maternal mortality rates in half. And here is what is even worse, maternal mortality disproportionately affects women of color. Pregnancy-related death is nearly four times higher among African American women. And there are multiple factors that contribute to these maternal mortality rates—the high incidence of preeclampsia, obstetric hemorrhaging, and mental health conditions.

Now to combat this trend, 33 states have established maternal mortality review committees. These panels bring together local healthcare professionals who collectively review individual maternal deaths and then target individual policy solutions towards them. The panels have been very effective. In California, for example, which established one in 2006, they have reduced their maternal mortality by more than 55 percent. And that is why what this bill does is it provides federal support for state-based maternal mortality review committees including for states, critically, that have not yet established these panels. It also promotes efforts to standardize data collection practices for maternal mortality which will help public health experts, researchers, and policymakers develop evidence-based solutions to address this crisis.

The bill has 171 co-sponsors and a number of organizations, some which are here in the audience today. The March of Dimes, the American College of Obstetrics and Gynecologists, and others all support it and so I really hope we can quickly advance the bill. I hope we can pass it by the end of the year and send it to the President's desk. Thank you and I yield back.

Mr. BURGESS. The chair thanks the gentlelady. The gentlelady yields back and this concludes with member opening statements. The chair would remind all members that pursuant to committee rules, members' opening statements will be made part of the record.

We do want to thank our witness on the first panel for being here today and taking time to testify before the subcommittee.

I do want, as a housekeeping note, after Representative Herrera Beutler testifies we will move immediately to the second panel. We will not break in between the panels of witnesses. And again as is the custom, when we have a Member at the witness table there will not be questions from the dais to the Member, so we will go right into the second panel after Representative Herrera Beutler testifies.

So our first witness is Representative Herrera Beutler from the State of Washington who is principal author of this legislation. We appreciate you being here today and you are recognized 5 minutes for your opening statement, please.

STATEMENT OF HON. JAIME HERRERA BEUTLER, A REPRESENTATIVE IN CONGRESS FROM THE STATE OF WASHINGTON

Ms. HERRERA BEUTLER. Thank you, Mr. Chairman, for having this hearing and for your work in this field. This isn't an issue of the moment for you, but this is what you have dedicated your life to and we are very grateful.

Thank you, Ranking Member Green, for your support of this critical issue, and members of the subcommittee today for participating in this effort to reduce maternal mortality in the United States and for giving me this opportunity to speak in strong support of this discussion draft of the Preventing Maternal Mortality Deaths Act that is before us.

So you either are a mom or you have a mom, so this issue impacts you. The very title of this bill speaks to why I have introduced this bipartisan legislation with my co-sponsor Ms. DeGette from Colorado. We have to take vital steps towards moving this bill in Congress and I believe we are going to save lives and prevent more families from suffering the profound loss of a cherished family member.

The testimonies today will shed light on a truly disturbing trend in our nation. More mothers die from pregnancy-related or pregnancy-associated deaths here in the U.S. than in any developed country in the world. Although the assumption is often that a nation with some of the most advanced obstetric and emergency care would also demonstrate low maternal mortality rates, tragically, an estimated 700–900 maternal deaths occur in the U.S. every year.

And not only does the U.S. rank 47th for maternal mortality globally, we have actually seen an increase in maternal deaths in recent years. This makes us one of only eight nations in the world with rising maternal mortality rates. It is unacceptable. In fact, Iran has a better maternal mortality rate than we do here in the United States.

In New Jersey where Mr. Pallone is from, and he knows this, if you are a woman of color, a black woman, out of 100,000 deaths, 79 are likely to pass away from a pregnancy-associated or pregnancy-related death. You are three or four times more likely as a woman of color to experience this tragedy in our country. It is unacceptable. For families, single fathers, grandparents, and children who have all lost a mother, perhaps the most heart-wrenching of all of this is that according to the CDC 60 percent of these maternal deaths could have been prevented.

As a mother, as a citizen, and a lawmaker, I believe we can and we must do better. It is time for this to become a national priority, which is why I am proud to speak in support of the Preventing Maternal Deaths Act. This legislation would enable states to establish and strengthen maternal mortality review committees. MMRCs bring together local experts in maternal, infant, and public health to review each and every instance of a pregnancy-related or pregnancy-associated death. We are going to investigate every single one because these moms are worth it. This is going to give us the information to understand why it is happening and what we need to do to fix it. This is how we are going to save future mothers' lives.

As members of the committee are aware, we know many of the conditions that contribute to high maternal mortality rate such as preeclampsia, gestational diabetes, obstetric hemorrhage, as well as emerging challenges such as suicide and substance use disorder. However, the truth is that the available data is woefully inadequate, which greatly hinders our ability to understand why mothers are dying. The Preventing Maternal Deaths Act seeks to address this data deficiency by empowering states to participate in national information sharing through the CDC, allowing for increased collaboration and the development of best practices.

Now before closing, I want to note that the legislation before us was crafted from key policy recommendations made by multiple organizations supporting this bill including the Association of Maternal & Child Health Programs, the American College of Obstetricians and Gynecologists, the March of Dimes, Preeclampsia Foundation, the Society for Maternal-Fetal Medicine—thank you to all of you tireless warriors in this fight.

Finally, and most importantly, I would like to extend my deepest gratitude to the families, fathers—one of whom you are going to hear from today, sitting behind me. Charles Johnson is going to tell you the story of the preventable death of his hero and hopefully this will be a tribute to ending those tragedies. He wants no one else to go through what he has gone through.

And to every advocate who has spoken out, shared their stories, and called for change, these courageous individuals are the champions of this movement and this bill. With wide bipartisan support and well over a 160 cosponsors in the House, I remain committed to passing the Preventing Maternal Deaths Act into law and I look forward to working with this committee, you, Mr. Chairman, and my colleagues in Congress to accomplish this imperative goal.

With that I thank you and I yield back.

[The prepared statement of Ms. Herrera Beutler follows:]

U.S. House of Representatives Energy and Commerce Committee, Subcommittee on Health Hearing: "Better Data and Better Outcomes: Reducing Maternal Mortality in the U.S." Testimony of: Congresswoman Jaime Herrera Beutler September 27, 2018

Thank you Chairman Burgess, Ranking Member Green, and Members of the Subcommittee for holding this hearing on reducing maternal mortality in the United States and for this opportunity to speak in strong support of the discussion draft of the *Preventing Maternal Deaths Act* that is before us.

The very title of this bill speaks to why I have introduced this bipartisan legislation and to why we are here today. We are here to take vital steps toward moving a bill in Congress that I believe will save lives and prevent more families from suffering the profound loss of a mother.

The testimonies today will shed light on a truly disturbing trend in our nation – more mothers die from pregnancy-related or pregnancy-associated causes here in the U.S. than *any* other developed country in the world.

Although the assumption is often that a nation with some of the most advanced obstetric and emergency care would also demonstrate low maternal mortality rates, tragically, an estimated 700 - 900 maternal deaths occur in the U.S. every year. Not only does the U.S. rank 47th for maternal mortality globally, we have actually seen an *increase* in maternal deaths in recent years. This makes us one of only eight nations in the world with *rising* maternal mortality rates.

For the families, single fathers, grandparents, and children who have lost a mother, perhaps the most heart-wrenching of all is that the Centers for Disease Control and Prevention estimates that *60 percent* of these maternal deaths could have been prevented.

As a mother, a citizen, and a lawmaker, I believe that we can and must do better. It is time for this to become a national priority, which is why I am proud to speak in support of the Preventing Maternal Deaths Act.

This legislation would enable states to establish or strengthen maternal mortality review committees. MMRCs bring together local experts in maternal, infant, and public health to review each and every instance of a pregnancy-related or pregnancy-associated death in order to understand what went wrong and how to save future mothers' lives.

As Members of the Committee are aware, we know of many conditions that contribute to high maternal mortality rates, such as preeclampsia, gestational diabetes, obstetric hemorrhage, as well as emerging challenges such as suicide and substance use disorder. However, the truth is that the available data is woefully inadequate, which greatly hinders our ability to understand why mothers are dying.

The Preventing Maternal Deaths Act seeks to address this data deficiency by empowering states to participate in national information sharing through the CDC, allowing for increased collaboration and the development of best practices.

Before closing, I would like to note that the legislation before us was crafted from key policy recommendations made by multiple organizations that are supporting this bill - including the Association of Maternal & Child Health Programs, the American College of Obstetricians and Gynecologists, March of Dimes, Preeclampsia Foundation, and the Society for Maternal-Fetal Medicine.

Finally, and most importantly, I would like to extend my deepest gratitude to the families, fathers, and advocates who have spoken out, shared their stories, and called for change. These courageous individuals are the champions of this movement and this bill.

With wide bipartisan support and over 160 cosponsors in the House, I remain committed to passing Preventing Maternal Deaths Act into law and I look forward to working with the Committee and my colleagues in Congress to accomplish this imperative goal.

Thank you.

Mr. BURGESS. We thank you, Representative Herrera Beutler, for, number one, putting forward the discussion draft and working on it so hard over this past year in bringing all of the different people together that had to finally come together to get this hearing a reality today. And I know it took a lot of work on your part and we really appreciate your dedication. So thank for being with us this morning and we will move immediately to our second panel.

And while the transition is occurring, I will just use this time to thank all of our witnesses for being here today and taking time to testify before the subcommittee. Each witness will be given the opportunity to deliver an opening statement followed by questions from members.

Mr. GREEN. Mr. Chairman?

Mr. BURGESS. For what purpose does the gentleman from Texas seek recognition?

Mr. GREEN. I would like to submit the following letters, ask unanimous consent to submit the following letters for the record. From the Moms Rising, Alexis Joy Foundation, and the Society for Maternal Fetal Medicine into the record.

Mr. BURGESS. Without objection, so ordered.

[The information appears at the conclusion of the hearing.

Mr. BURGESS. Do we have copies of those?

Mr. GREEN. Yes.

Mr. BURGESS. So today we are going to hear from Mr. Charles Johnson, founder of 4Kira4Moms; Ms. Stacey Stewart, president of the March of Dimes; Dr. Lynne Coslett-Charlton, Pennsylvania District Legislative Chair, The American College of Obstetricians and Gynecologists; and Dr. Joia Crear Perry, president of the National Birth Equity Collaborative. We appreciate each of you being here today.

And Mr. Johnson, you are now recognized 5 minutes for an opening statement. Please turn your microphone on. Pull it close. This is the premier technology committee in the United States House of Representatives and we have fairly rudimentary amplification devices.

So Mr. Johnson, you are recognized.

Statements of Charles S. Johnson, IV, Founder, 4Kira4Moms; Stacey D. Stewart, President, March of Dimes; Lynne Coslett-Charlton, MD, Pennsylvania District Legislative Chair, the American College of Obstetricians and Gynecologists; and, Joia Crear Perry, MD, Founder and President, National Birth Equity Collaborative

Statement of Charles Johnson

Mr. JOHNSON. I think I will manage. Thank you so much. So, first and foremost, to members of this committee, thank you. It is an honor to be here speaking on behalf of the tens of thousands of families that have been affected by this maternal mortality crisis and hundreds of thousands of women who have been affected by near misses.

So let me just begin by telling you about the woman that absolutely changed my life. My wife, Kira Dixon Johnson, was the closest thing that I had ever met to a superhero. She made me far better than I ever thought I could be and she was far better than I ever deserved. We are talking about a woman that ran marathons; that raced cars; that spoke five languages fluently.

So we were blessed to welcome our first son, Charles, on September 18th of 2014. We always wanted back-to-back boys, Chairman Burgess, and we were blessed to find out we were going to welcome our second son, Langston, in April of 2016. We walked into Cedars-Sinai Medical Center on April 12th of 2016 with a woman that just wasn't in good health, she was in exceptional health. This picture that you see on the screen is literally taken 10 days before Kira went in for the procedure.

We went in for what was supposed to be a routine scheduled C-section on what was supposed to be the happiest day of our lives and we walked right into what was a nightmare. Shortly after the procedure took place around 2 o'clock, shortly afterwards we went back to recovery. As I am sitting there reflecting in all this glow and pride of being a new father for the second time, Kira is resting, my new baby is resting, and as I look at her bedside I begin to see the catheter begin to turn red with blood.

I brought it to the attention of the staff, the nurses at Cedars-Sinai. They came in. They said we are going to do a couple of things. We are going to order a set of tests and we are going to order a CT scan to be performed stat. I was concerned, but I said you know what, my wife is healthy and we are at what is supposed to be one of the best hospitals in the world. I am concerned but we have got a plan, OK.

Blood work comes back, it is showing that it is abnormal and she is hemorrhaging and they ordered a CT scan that was supposed to be performed stat. Keep in mind this is around 4 o'clock. 5 o'clock comes, no CT scan. Her blood level was continuing to drop. By this time she is beginning to shiver uncontrollably. 6 o'clock and no CT scan. She is beginning to become pale, she is in extreme pain. 7 o'clock, 8 o'clock comes, no CT scan. I am begging, I am pleading the staff to do something.

And around 9 o'clock as I continue to plea for my wife's life, the staff at Cedars-Sinai Medical Center tells me, sir, your wife just isn't a priority right now. 8 o'clock comes, 9 o'clock, 10 o'clock. They said, well, we need to do a blood transfusion. I am saying, well, where is the CT scan? It wasn't until after midnight that they finally took my wife back to surgery, after I begged and pleaded for them to take action for more than 10 hours. When they took Kira back to surgery they opened her up and there were three and a half liters of blood in her abdomen and she coded immediately.

Now I am here to tell you this. I am not here to tell you what I think. I am here to tell you what I know. There are people on this panel that are far more intelligent than I will ever be that are going to talk to you about the statistics and how horrifying they are. What I am here to tell you is this. That there is no statistic that can quantify what it is like to tell an 18-month-old that his mother is never coming home. There is no matrices that can quantify what it is like to explain to a son that will never know his mother just how amazing she was.

My wife deserved better. Women all over this country deserve better. I am so grateful to my shero, Congresswoman Jaime Herrera Beutler. Thank you so much, Congresswoman DeGette. And for those of you all who have supported this bill, I honest to goodness would love to come up there and just give you a big hug, but I have been explained that that is not protocol.

And let me say this for those that choose to stand in opposition of this bill, you don't owe me an explanation. You owe an explanation to my boys. You owe Tara Hansen's son an explanation. You owe Mustafa Shabazz and his son an explanation. We have an opportunity to do something, here and now, to send a loud, definitive message to this country that women and babies matter.

Lastly, Kira and I always talked about raising men that would change the world. It is time for us to stop telling our children that they can change the world and show them how it is done. Thank you for your time.

[The prepared statement of Mr. Johnson follows:]

September 24, 2018

TESTIMONY OF CHARLES JOHNSON IV, HUSBAND OF THE LATE KIRA JOHNSON, FOUNDER OF 4KIRA4MOMS, ADVOCATE FOR IMPROVED MATERNAL HEALTH POLICIES, BEFORE THE SUBCOMMITTEE ON HEALTH, COMMITTEE ON ENERGY AND COMMERCE, U.S. HOUSE OF REPRESENTATIVES, "BETTER DATA AND BETTER OUTCOMES: REDUCING MATERNAL MORTALITY IN THE U.S."

9:15 a.m., Thursday, September 27th, 2018

Good Morning Mr. Chairman, Ranking Member Green, members of the committee: my name is Charles Johnson the IV. I'd like to thank the committee for inviting me to testify today on H.R. 1318: Preventing Maternal Deaths Act of 2017. I have envisioned the opportunity to speak before this committee for some time now and could not be more grateful than to share my family's story with you today.

I have just introduced myself to you in my opening statement as Charles Johnson the IV, however, these days I am known as "Charles and Langston's Dad." Following the esteemed title of Dad, is that of "Kira's husband."

I met Kira several times before we connected. Trying to catch Kira's attention was like trying to catch a butterfly. Kira was the most amazing person I have ever met. She spoke four different languages, lived in China and had run several companies. Her idea of a relaxing date was skydiving...her idea of a romantic date was drag racing. I was smitten with her zest for life- her enthusiasm- I couldn't wait to see what was going to happen next. We got married in a surprise destination wedding, one which I took pains to make sure I made an impressive impact on my bride, like she made on me every day. It was a dream come true: our wedding, our honeymoon, our new life as a married couple, the start of our new family. We had the rest our lives in front of us! Nothing could stop us.

On April 12, 2016 my life partner, my best friend and amazing Mom, Kira lost her life after a routine scheduled C-section at Cedars Sinai delivering our 2nd son, Langston Johnson. Kira had delivered our first son, Charles V, via cesarean section, so we were both prepared for the process, procedure and recovery. After delivering another perfect baby, I was sitting next to Kira by her bedside in the recovery room. That is when I first noticed blood in her catheter. I notified staff immediately. A series of test were ordered. Along with a CT scan to be performed "STAT." I understood "STAT" to mean the CT scan would be performed immediately. Hours passed and Kira's symptoms escalated throughout the rest of the afternoon and into the evening. We were told by the medical staff at Cedars Sinai Kira was not a priority and we waited for her CT scan to be done...we waited for the hospital to act so she could begin her recovery. Kira kept telling me, "Charles, I'm so cold; Charles, I don't feel right." She repeated these same words to me for several hours. After more than 10 hours of waiting. After 10 hours of watching my wife's condition deteriorate. After 10 hours of watching Kira suffer in excruciating pain needlessly. After 10 hours of begging and pleading them to help her. The medical staff at Cedars Sinai finally took action. As they prepared Kira for surgery, I was holding her hand as we walked down the hall to the operating room. Kira looked at me and said, "Baby, I'm scared." I told her, without doubt, everything was going to be fine. The doctor told me I would see her in 15 minutes. Kira was wheeled into surgery and it was discovered that she had massive internal bleeding caused by horrible medical negligence that occurred during her routine C-section. She had approximately 3 litters of blood in her abdomen. Kira died at 2:22 a.m. April 17, 2016. Langston was 11 hours old.

As someone who experienced firsthand what it is like to have your spouse die in front of you, I do not have the words to describe the loss my family has suffered. My boys no longer have their Mother. Kira was the most amazing role model and Mother any boy could ever wish to have. I no longer have the love of my life; my best friend.

I vowed that I would take this tragedy and turn it into a mission fueled by the memory of Kira and the passion she brought to life every day. I have taken my grief and found peace by tirelessly working on maternal health and maternal outcomes. I am the founder of 4Kira4Moms. 4Kira4Moms mission to advocate for improved maternal health policies and regulations, to educate the public about the impact of maternal mortality in communities, provide peer support to the victim's family, friends, and promote the idea that maternal mortality should be viewed, and discussed, as a human rights issue. My Kira lost her life, and I simply could not believe that her death, my family's experience, was not an anomaly. My situation and my family are not unique. The maternal mortality rate is rising in the United States. According to the Lancet, 26.7 women out of 100,000 die directly as a direct result of maternal mortality. Maternal mortality figures have been rising exponentially in the United States over the past 2 decades. In 1990, the US had 674 recorded maternal mortality deaths per 100K; by 2015, the number had risen to 1063 women per 100K. Women of color, regardless of income or education, are dying at a rate of 3 to 4 times higher. My wife is now a 2017 maternal mortality rate statistic.

Each maternal death is equal to approximately 70 mothers experience a "near miss," meaning they almost die. Based on CDC figures, approximately 50K mothers almost died from childbirth as recent at 2014. This has to stop!

I'm here today because the committee wanted to hear my story, Kira's story, Charles and Langston's story. The importance of passing H.R. 1318: Preventing Maternal Mortality Act of 2017 is part of that story. This country deserves to know why our mothers are dying. Women and families who want to bear children should know what leads to maternal mortality, and "near misses." I want to help everyone out there who wishes to someday become a parent, the most blessed gift in the world, and every provider who helps those amazing women bring life into the world, to understand what to look for; how to help, when to listen.

Thank you for the opportunity to hear my testimony today. The time is now for political will to address a situation that chose me without any knowledge. HR 1318: Preventing Maternal Mortality Act of 2017 will assist states to give us the knowledge on why our country's Mothers are dying and how to help put an end to such tragedy. That knowledge may have saved Kira's life.

ADDENDUM

- 4Moms4Kira Campaign
- How Judge Hatchett's Son Is Coping After His Wife's Childbirth Death: 'I Take It Day by Day'
- Maternal Mortality: an American Crisis
- Too many mothers are dying after childbirth. A hospital hopes to save them.
- Charles Johnson shares Kira's story at the March for Moms Washington DC. https://www.youtube.com/watch?v=05uBCBfrY4g

Attached: copy of Johnson family complaint for damages. Outlining the timeline of the events that lead to Kira Johnson's death.

Attached: photos of Kira Dixon

Michael L. Oran, Esq. (SBN: 110970)
LAW OFFICES OF MICHAEL L. ORAN
801 South Grand Avenue
11th Floor
Los Angeles, California 90071
TEL: (213) 624-1177
FAX: (213) 624-1161
EMAIL: miloran@mloesq.com

Attorneys for Plaintiffs

CONFORMED COPY
ORIGINAL FILED
Superior Court of California
County of Los Angeles
MAR 22 2017
Sherri R. Carter, Executive Officer/Clerk
By: [signature], Deputy
Moses Soto

SUPERIOR COURT OF THE STATE OF CALIFORNIA

FOR THE COUNTY OF LOS ANGELES

CHARLES JOHNSON, IV; CHARLES JOHNSON, V, a minor, by and through his Guardian ad Litem, CHARLES JOHNSON, IV; LANGSTON JOHNSON, a minor, by and through his Guardian ad Litem, CHARLES JOHNSON, IV, Plaintiffs, vs. CEDARS-SINAI MEDICAL CENTER, a business organization, form unknown; ARJANG NAIM, M.D.; KATHRYN SHARMA, M.D.; SARA CHURCHILL, M.D.; STUART MARTIN, M.D.; BENHAM KASHANCHI, M.D.; and DOES 1 to 100, Inclusive, Defendants.	CASE NO. BC 655107 **COMPLAINT FOR DAMAGES:** **(1) Wrongful Death** **(2) Negligent Infliction of Emotional Distress**

Plaintiffs Charles Johnson, IV, Charles Johnson, V, a minor, by and through his Guardian ad Litem, Charles Johnson, IV, and Langston Johnson, a minor, by and through his Guardian ad Litem, Charles Johnson, IV, allege as follows:

///

///

1

COMPLAINT FOR DAMAGES

FIRST CAUSE OF ACTION FOR WRONGFUL DEATH BY PLAINTIFFS CHARLES JOHNSON, IV, CHARLES JOHNSON, V and LANGSTON JOHNSON AGAINST ALL DEFENDANTS

1. Kyira Adele Dixon was born on June 26, 1976. Kyira was married to Charles Johnson, IV. Their first son, Charles Johnson, V, was born on September 18, 2014 by primary cesarean section delivery. Plaintiff Charles Johnson, IV had been present at the cesarean section delivery of his first son. Kyira Adele Dixon was a healthy, vibrant, fun, loving wife and mother.

2. In 2015, Kyira became pregnant again. She, her husband and son relocated to Los Angeles to pursue business and other opportunities. Once here, her pre-natal care was transferred to Defendant Benham Kashanchi, M.D. Defendant Benham Kashanchi, M.D. followed her through her pre-natal care. However, before her planned elective cesarean section, her care was transferred to Defendant Arjang Naim, M.D. Both Defendants Arjang Naim, M.D. and Benham Kashanchi, M.D. were in the Defendant Cedars-Sinai Medical Center's operative suite at the time of the delivery described herein.

3. The facts leading up to the death of Kyira Adele Dixon taken from the medical records, and with approximate times, include, but are not limited to, the following:

(A) Kyira was 39 years-old;

(B) Kyira, accompanied by her husband, Plaintiff Charles Johnson, IV, presented to Defendant Cedars-Sinai Hospital on April 12, 2016 at approximately 12:30 p.m. for a repeat elective cesarean delivery. The delivery was performed by Defendant Arjang Naim, M.D. and assisted by Defendant Benham Kashanchi,

M.D. Plaintiff Charles Johnson, IV, was present in the operating room;

(C) Kyira was taken to the operative suite at 2:00 p.m. A foley catheter was inserted at 2:15 p.m. The delivery started at 2:31 p.m. Langston Johnson was born at 2:33 p.m. The procedure was completed at or about 2:48 p.m. At 3:00 p.m., Kyira was out of the operating room and taken to the Post Anesthesia Care Unit (PACU). Plaintiff Charles Johnson, IV, continued to be present with his wife. At 3:04 p.m. Kyira was "skin to skin" bonding with their baby;

(D) At 4:45 p.m., Kyira's fundus[1] had risen from +2 to +4 cms above the umbilicus. This may be associated with failure of the uterus to contract after delivery, a condition called uterine atony. Atony can lead to or be a symptom of a potentially life-threatening condition known as postpartum hemorrhage;

(E) Shortly before 5:00 p.m., blood tinged urine was seen in Kyira's foley catheter;

(F) By 5:24 p.m., Kyira's foley catheter was draining bright red blood. The records indicate that a resident physician was called by a nurse "to evaluate the rising fundus and concern for excessive bleeding.";

(G) Shortly thereafter, the foley catheter was removed for "bloody urine." It was replaced at 5:30 p.m. Defendant Dr. Naim was made aware of his patient Kyira's situation;

///

///

[1] The fundus is the upper rounded extremity of the uterus above the openings of the uterine tubes.

(H) At 5:38 p.m., Kyira's fundus continued to be at +4 and frank red blood was still present and seen in Kyira's foley catheter;

(I) 7 minutes later Kyira's foley catheter was draining "complete red blood." A bedside ultrasound showed a 6 cm (2.3 inches) heterogenous fluid collection posterior to bladder/ anterior to uterus compressing the bladder suspicious for large hematoma[2]. Uterotonics, Pitocin and Cytotec, were ordered for apparent uterine atony;

(J) Defendant Dr. Naim was again notified;

(K) Kyira was given Dilaudid for pain. She was also given an intravenous fluid bolus of 500 ml.;

(L) At 6:12 p.m., labs were ordered. Kyira's results showed:

- White Blood Count abnormal at 19.1 (normal range: 4-11 1000 UL);
- Red Blood Count abnormal at 3.01 (normal range: 3.6-5.11);
- Hemoglobin abnormal at 9.2 (normal range 12-16.0 G/dl); and
- Hematocrit abnormal at 27% (normal range 36-47%).

In addition, the records reflect that Dr. Kashanchi also ordered a separate hemoglobin and hematocrit blood test. The results showed:

- Hemoglobin abnormal at 9.2; and
- Hematocrit abnormal at 27%.

---

[2] A hematoma is a mass or abnormal collection of clotted blood within the tissues.

A fibrinogen[3] blood test at about the same time showed a result of 228 which is on the low end of normal (normal range is 200-400 mg/dl);

(M) At 6:44 p.m., a "stat" CT of Kyira's abdomen and pelvis and CT urogram were ordered by Stuart Martin, M.D. The records indicate the "reason for stat/expedite: surgical emergency." The records also document that Kyira had "intractable" abdominal pain and frank blood per foley catheter. The order comments also state: "Please add imaging, i.e. CT abd/pelvis with IV contrast as needed to fully evaluate the patient's post op abdomen and pelvis; high concern for pelvic hematoma but uncertain regarding injury to bladder and ureters.";

(N) Kyira's bleeding continued. At 7:13 p.m., Dr. Sharma noted that Kyira had not had any urine output after 5:00 p.m. Dr. Sharma performed another ultrasound. It showed the hematoma had enlarged. Kyira and her husband were told that although the hematoma appeared "stable" there was concern regarding the "blood in foley with little to no urine output. Will obtain STAT imaging of pelvis and lower urinary tract to ensure integrity...". Dr. Naim was made aware;

(O) More fluids were provided via IV infusion. Labs reported between 7:35 and 8:01 showed:

- White Blood Count abnormal at 21.5;
- Red Blood Count abnormal at 2.58;

///

---

[3] Fibrinogen is a protein in the plasma that originates in the liver. It is converted to fibrin during the blood clotting process (coagulation).

- Hemoglobin abnormal at 7.6;
- Hematocrit abnormal at 23.7%; and
- Fibrinogen abnormal at 186.

(P) At 8:00 p.m., Kyira was seen by Dr. Churchill. She had still only produced little to no urine despite having been given fluids. There was still blood in her foley catheter. Kyira's hemoglobin and hematocrit were noted as continuing to drop and her heart rate was tachycardic.[4] The estimated blood loss was about 1500 cc's. "This suggests symptomatic acute blood loss anemia and decision made to proceed with 2 units of PRBC" [packed red blood cells]. "Proceeding also with CT urogram to evaluate kidneys/ureters/bladder given frank blood in foley"; Kyira's situation was discussed with Dr. Naim and Dr. Sharma;

(Q) Although packed red blood cells were started at 8:41 p.m., plasma, which provides blood clotting proteins including fibrinogen, was not ordered until 11:21 p.m.;

R) At 8:47 p.m. the records document that Dr. Naim was at the bedside examining Kyira in the PACU. Dr. Naim knew at that time that Kyira continued with "bloody urine," had an abnormal hemoglobin of 7, that her heart rate was consistent with tachycardia and that she had a "possible hematoma.";

(S) At just about 9:00 p.m., Kyira was holding her baby in the PACU where she had remained and still had not been transferred to post partum;

///

///

---

[4] Tachycardia is a resting heart rate of at least 100 beats per minute.

(T) At 10:44 p.m., that the CT scans that had been ordered "stat" 4 hours earlier still had not been done. In fact the records do not reflect these scans were ever performed;

(U) At 10:55 pm the nurse notified the doctors that Kyira's blood pressures were in the 70's/50's. Dr. Churchill and another doctor were at the bedside to assess Kyira. Even after changing the blood pressure cuff, Kyira's blood pressure was 82/53;

(V) At approximately 11:25 p.m., Dr. Naim was notified with a concern "for active internal bleeding." Despite blood in the foley, no urine output, abnormal labs, symptoms suggesting acute blood loss, enlarging hematoma, it was not until approximately 11:30 p.m. and thereafter that a surgical discussion was held and consent provided for surgery;

(W) At 11:42 p.m., Dr. Churchill and Dr. Sharma were at the bedside. Kyira felt "a little more groggy then before", her heart rate was 120 at rest and her blood pressure was 90/70. Dr. Sharma performed a repeat ultrasound. The ultrasound "found expanding hematoma and now free fluid." Dr. Sharma and Dr. Churchill recommended taking Kyira to surgery to identify the source of the bleeding. Yet Dr. Naim, who was also at the bedside at this time, and in the face of these abnormal findings as previously set forth, wished "to continue expectant management at this time.";

(X) Shortly thereafter, the massive transfusion protocol was initiated on Kyira. Massive Transfusion Protocol means packed red blood cells, platelets and plasma given in "massive" quantities to support circulation and coagulation during massive hemorrhage;

(Y) Kyira was taken to surgery around 12:30 a.m. on April 13, 2016. During surgery Kyira was found to have 3 liters of blood in her abdomen;

(Z) Kyira did not survive the ongoing massive blood loss. Kyira was pronounced dead at 2:22 a.m. on April 13, 2016; and

(AA) The autopsy stated that the cause of "death was due to hemorrhagic shock, due to acute hemoperitoneum," status post cesarean section.

4. The surviving heirs of Kyira Adele Dixon, deceased (hereinafter referred to as "decedent") are Charles Johnson, IV (husband), Charles Johnson, V (son) and Langston Johnson (son). There are no other heirs that Plaintiffs are aware of.

5. Defendants DOES 1 through 10, inclusive, are potential heirs of decedent and entitled to bring this action pursuant to C.C.P. Section 377.60, and they are named as Defendants in this action as their true names and capacities as potential heirs are presently unknown to Plaintiffs herein.

6. The true names, identities or capacities, whether individual, associate, corporate or otherwise of Defendants DOES 11 through 100, inclusive, are unknown to plaintiffs who therefore sue said defendants by such fictitious names. When the true names, identities, or capacities of such fictitiously designated defendants are ascertained, Plaintiffs will ask leave of court to amend this Complaint to insert the true names, identities and capacities together with the charging allegations.

7. At all times herein mentioned, Defendants and each of them, were the agents, servants, employees and joint venturers of each other and of their said codefendants, and were acting within

8

COMPLAINT FOR DAMAGES

the purpose and scope of their employment, agency or joint venture.

8. Plaintiffs are informed and believe and thereon allege that each of the Defendants sued herein as a DOE (except DOES 1 through 10, inclusive) is responsible in some manner for the events or happenings herein referred to, thereby proximately causing the injuries and damages to their decedent Kyira as herein alleged.

9. That all of the facts, acts, events and circumstances herein mentioned and described occurred in the County of Los Angeles, State of California.

10. That at all times herein mentioned, Defendants Arjang Naim, M.D., Kathryn Sharma, M.D., Sara Churchill, M.D., Stuart Martin, M.D., Benham Kashanchi, M.D. and DOES 11 through 30, inclusive, were and now are physicians and surgeons, holding themselves out as duly licensed to practice their professions under and by virtue of the laws of the State of California, and were and now are engaged in the practice of their professions in the State of California.

11. At all times mentioned herein, Defendants Arjang Naim, M.D., Kathryn Sharma, M.D., Sara Churchill, M.D., Stuart Martin, M.D., Benham Kashanchi, M.D. and DOES 11 through 30, inclusive, held themselves out to the public at large and to Plaintiffs herein as qualified physicians and surgeons duly licensed to practice their professions by virtue and under the laws of the State of California, with expertise, specialized knowledge, training, education, learning skill, techniques and expertise in certain specialities of medicine.

12. That holding themselves out as experts and specialists in specialized fields of surgery and medicine, possessing skills, learning and experience in said specialties, Defendants herein, at all times mentioned herein, represented to Plaintiffs that they would, at all times, exercise and use skill, prudence, learning and experience in said specialties. Defendants herein, at all times mentioned herein, represented to Plaintiffs that they would at all times exercise and use the skill, prudence, learning, knowledge and expertise in the care and treatment of decedent in accordance with the standard of practice among competent, reputable and prudent physicians practicing their specialties in the State of California.

13. At all times herein mentioned, Defendants Arjang Naim, M.D., Kathryn Sharma, M.D., Sara Churchill, M.D., Stuart Martin, M.D., Benham Kashanchi, M.D. and DOES 11 through 30, inclusive, held themselves out to the public at large and to Plaintiffs as duly qualified physicians and surgeons, duly licensed to practice their profession by virtue of and under the laws of the State of California, and exercising prudence, reasonable judgment and care in the selection, employment and control of qualified, trained, experienced nurses, nursing personnel, assistants, aides and employees, performing services and caring for patients, including, but limited to decedent, under their supervision, control, direction, responsibility and authority.

14. At all times herein mentioned, Defendants Cedars-Sinai Medical Center and DOES 31 through 50, inclusive, were business organizations, form unknown, organized and existing under the laws of the State of California.

15. At all times herein mentioned, Defendants Cedars-Sinai Medical Center and DOES 31 through 50, inclusive, were and at all times herein mentioned are, a partnership. Defendants DOES 11 through 20, inclusive, are, and at all times herein mentioned were, members of the foregoing named partnership and are sued herein individually and by said common name pursuant to the provisions C.C.P. Section 369.5.

16. At all times herein mentioned, Defendants DOES 51 through 60, inclusive, were and are registered nurses, nurse practitioners, licensed vocational nurses, practical nurses, registered technicians and other paramedical personnel, holding themselves out as duly licensed to practice their profession under and by virtue of the law of the State of California, and were and now are engaged in the practice of their profession under and by virtue of the laws of the State of California.

17. At all times herein mentioned, Defendants DOES 61 through 70, inclusive, were aides, attendants, technicians, nursing or medical students, acting as agents, employees or servants of some or all of the other defendants, within the course and scope of said agency or employment.

18. Defendants Cedars-Sinai Medical Center and DOES 71 through 80, inclusive, were at all times herein mentioned, duly organized California corporations and partnerships existing under and by virtue of the laws of the State of California. Said defendants, and each of them, owned, operated, managed, controlled and administered a general medical facility, hospital or 24-hour care facility within said County, State of California, and held themselves out to the public at large and to Plaintiffs

herein as properly equipped, fully accredited, competently staffed by qualified and prudent personnel and operating in compliance with the standard of care maintained in other properly equipped and efficiently operated and administered accredited general medical facilities, hospitals and outpatient clinics in said community, offering full, competent and efficient hospital, emergency, clinical, medical, surgical, laboratory, x-ray, anesthesia, paramedical services and outpatient clinics to the general public and to decedent herein. Plaintiffs are informed and believe and thereon allege that said defendants, and each of them, administered, governed, controlled, managed and directed all the necessary functions, activities and operations of said general medical facility, hospital or 24-hour care facility, including its nursing care, intern, resident and house staff, physicians and surgeons, medical staff, x-ray, intensive care, recovery room and emergency room departments and clinics, including but not limited to personnel, staff and supplies of said facilities and clinics.

19. Plaintiffs are informed and believe and upon such information and belief allege that at all times herein mentioned, Defendants, and each of them, were the agents, servants, employees and copartners of their said codefendants, and as such, were acting within the course and scope of such agency, partnership, and employment at all times herein mentioned; that each and every defendant, as aforesaid, when acting as a principal, was negligent in the selecting, hiring and maintaining of each and every other defendant, as its agents, servants, partners and employees.

20. At all times herein mentioned, Plaintiffs' decedent Kyira was in the exclusive custody and control of Defendants, and each of them.

21. Prior to April 13, 2016, decedent Kyira, who was pregnant, consulted defendants, and each of them, for the purpose of obtaining her medical care and treatment and employed defendants to care and do all things necessary in caring for her. Said Defendants undertook the employment and understood and agreed to diagnose, care and treat decedent and do all things necessary and proper in connection therewith, and said defendants, and each of them, thereafter entered into such employment, individually, and by and through their employees, employers and agents.

22. At all times herein mentioned, and prior and subsequent thereto Defendants Cedars-Sinai Medical Center and DOES 71 through 80, inclusive, and each of them, so negligently and carelessly failed to properly ensure the character, quality, ability and competence of individuals treating patients in said centers, hospitals and clinics, that Plaintiffs were caused to suffer and did suffer, the injuries and damages hereinafter alleged.

23. Plaintiffs name the defendants herein, and each of them, because plaintiffs are in doubt and do not know from which of said defendants plaintiffs are entitled to redress and whether the injuries and damages to the plaintiffs herein alleged were caused by the combined negligence of all of the defendants, or one or more of them. For that reason, Plaintiffs name all of said defendants and ask that the Court determine liability of

each and all of the said defendants in this action as to what extent and what responsibility falls upon each of said defendants either jointly or severally as may be found liable.

24. From and after said times, defendants, and each of them, so negligently examined decedent Kyira and diagnosed and failed to diagnose her condition and so negligently treated and cared for decedent while she was in the exclusive control of said defendants, and so negligently operated, managed, maintained, selected, designed, controlled and conducted their services, activities and equipment in connection with the care and treatment of decedent such that as a proximate result thereof, decedent Kyira died on April 13, 2016. The negligence of the Defendants, and each of them, includes, but is not limited to:

- Failing to appreciate and properly manage Kyira's post-partum hemorrhage in a timely manner;
- Failing to return Kyira to surgery in a timely manner;
- Among other acts and omissions.

25. Plaintiff Charles Johnson, IV is the husband of decedent Kyira and Plaintiffs Charles Johnson, V and Langston Johnson, are the sons of decedent Kyira.

26. At or about the time of the filing of this complaint, Charles Johnson, IV, the father of Plaintiffs Charles Johnson, V, a minor (DOB: 09/18/2014) and Langston Johnson, a minor (DOB: 04/12/2016), was appointed to serve as the Guardian Ad Litem for both Charles Johnson, V and Langston Johnson.

27. As a direct and proximate result of said negligence of the defendants and the death of decedent, Plaintiffs have been and will continue to be deprived of the love, companionship,

comfort, affection, society, solace, moral support, care, counsel, physical assistance, services, financial support and protection of decedent Kyira, and have thereby sustained pecuniary loss in a sum according to proof in the jurisdiction of this Court.

28. As a further, proximate result of the negligence of Defendants, and each of them, and the death of decedent, plaintiffs have incurred expenses for the funeral, cremation and/or burial of decedent Kyira, in a sum to be proven at the time of trial.

29. That prior to the filing of this action, three years had not elapsed from the date of the death, and a period of less than one calendar year had elapsed after Plaintiffs first learned, or had a reasonable opportunity to learn, of the fact that the injuries and death suffered and complained of herein were a proximate result of the negligent acts or omissions to act on the part of the Defendants.

SECOND CAUSE OF ACTION BY PLAINTIFF CHARLES JOHNSON, IV

FOR NEGLIGENT INFLICTION OF EMOTIONAL DISTRESS

30. Plaintiff repeats and realleges paragraphs 1, 2, 3, 6, 7, 8, 9, 10, 11, 12, 13, 14, 15, 16, 17, 18, 20, 21, 23, 24 and 29 of the allegations contained in the first cause of action as though each were set forth and incorporated herein in full.

31. At all times herein mentioned, Plaintiff Charles Johnson, IV was the lawfully wedded husband of decedent Kyira Adele Dixon.

///

///

32. Plaintiff Charles Johnson, IV was present and with his wife Kyira from the time she was admitted to give birth to their son until Kyira was taken to surgery on April 13, 2016.

33. Plaintiff Charles Johnson, IV was seated on the side of his wife where the bag collecting her urine was located. Plaintiff Charles Johnson, IV saw Kyira's foley catheter bag tinged with blood, saw the bag begin to turn red, called the red colored foley catheter bag to the attention of Kyira's nurses, saw the foley catheter bag get redder and redder with blood, saw the heightened activity of the health care staff as they became aware of the bright red blood in Kyira's foley catheter bag, saw the foley changed, and then again saw bright red blood fill Kyira's foley catheter bag, saw the health care staff perform an ultrasound on Kyira and state that there appeared to be a hematoma in her pelvis/abdomen, understood that a hematoma was a collection of blood, saw the health care providers perform another ultrasound and was advised that it still showed hematoma or blood clot, discussed with Kyira and her health care providers that the bright red blood in Kyira's foley catheter bag was "concerning" and due to Kyira actively bleeding, advised by the health care providers that a "stat" CT scans had been ordered and understood it was needed and necessary to identify the source of Kyira's bleeding, was advised by Kyira's health care providers that further confirmation of the fact that Kyira was continuing to actively bleed were her blood count values which were continuing to decline, asked why the "stat" CT scans ordered for Kyira and necessary to identify the source of her bleeding had not been performed, observed Kyira continue to get pale and

understood that Kyira's pallor was due to the continuing loss of blood, observed the health care providers provide Kyira with fluids and blood and understood that such fluids and blood was due to the Kyira's continuing loss of blood, repeatedly asked again why the "stat" CT scans ordered for Kyira and necessary to identify the source of her active bleeding, understood that despite the passage of hours since the bright red blood he observed in Kyira's foley catheter bag the health care providers had still not done anything to identify the source of the active bleeding and had not done anything to stop the active bleeding which he knew was continuing and causing Kyira's condition to continue to deteriorate, continued to express concern progressing to demanding information why his wife was continuing to deteriorate without any intervention improving her condition and continued to ask and then demand why the "stat" CT scans ordered for Kyira had not been done. The events described in this paragraph took place over approximately seven (7) hours.

34. Because of what he observed, what he heard and what he was told by the health care providers, Plaintiff Charles Johnson, IV, knew that Kyira's continued active bleeding caused a serious risk of harm to her. Because of what he observed, what he heard and what he knew, Plaintiff Charles Johnson, IV, was contemporaneously aware and understood that the inadequate actions of the health care providers over a period of approximately seven (7) hours were causing harm to Kyira because the source of her active bleeding had not been identified, the bleeding had not stopped, Kyira's condition was deteriorating to the point where she was experiencing pain, Kyira was pale and

groggy, and Kyira had and was continuing to lose blood which the health care providers were unable to sufficiently replace with fluids and blood products.

35. As a direct and proximate result of the failure of the Defendants to properly and timely respond to his wife's symptoms and the inadequate treatment provided to her by defendants, and each of them, Plaintiff Charles Johnson, IV did suffer serious and severe emotional disturbance, distress and shock and injury to his nervous system, all of which has caused, and continues to cause, and will cause in the future, serious mental and emotional suffering, in an amount in excess of the minimum jurisdiction of this court.

WHEREFORE, Plaintiffs pray for judgment against the Defendants, and each of them, as follows:

FOR THE FIRST AND SECOND CAUSES OF ACTION:

1. General damages according to proof;
2. Special damages according to proof;
3. Funeral and burial expenses according to proof;
4. Prejudgment interest;
5. For all costs of suit herein incurred; and
6. For such other and further relief as the Court may deem just and proper.

DATED: March 20, 2017 LAW OFFICES OF MICHAEL L. ORAN

BY: [signature]
MICHAEL L. ORAN, ESQ.
Attorneys for Plaintiffs
CHARLES JOHNSON, IV,
CHARLES JOHNSON, V and
LANGSTON JOHNSON

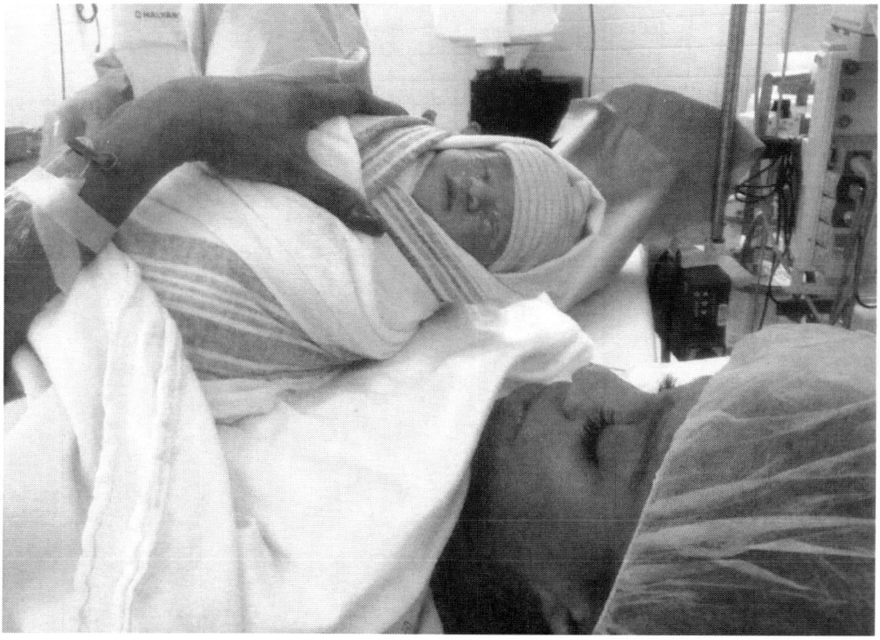

Mr. BURGESS. Mr. Johnson, we do sincerely appreciate your testimony and as a committee I will say we are terribly sorry for your loss, but grateful for your courage to be here today and present your testimony to us. Thank you, Mr. Johnson.

Ms. Stewart, you are recognized for 5 minutes.

STATEMENT OF STACEY STEWART

Ms. STEWART. Thank you, Mr. Chairman.

Mr. BURGESS. I know, he is tough to follow.

Ms. STEWART. Very hard to follow that so—and I am known by my family to be one of the biggest crybabies, but it is for good reason.

So thank you for inviting me to testify at this very important hearing today. I am Stacey Stewart. I am President of the March of Dimes. March of Dimes is leading the fight for the health of all moms and babies. And I would like everyone in this room to take a look at this blanket. Just about everyone that has had a child will never forget the very moment when a doctor placed a precious baby boy or baby girl into our arms wrapped into one of these blankets.

More than 700 times a year, beautiful babies are wrapped into these blankets, in one just like this one, but unfortunately there is no mother to hold a child that is wrapped in that blanket. So that is not just a statistic. There are 700 mothers that die every single year and almost and over 50,000 who experience dangerous complications that could have killed them, making the U.S. the most dangerous place in the developed world to give birth.

And we think and we know that you agree that this situation is completely unacceptable. Our nation is in the midst of a crisis of maternal and child health. Across this nation, virtually every measure of the health of pregnant women, new mothers, and infants is going in the wrong direction. The number of babies born premature is rising in this country. In many communities, infant mortality, rates of infant mortality exceed those in developing nations. Nations such as Slovenia and French Polynesia have better infant mortality rates than here in the United States.

Women are tragically dying, women like Kira, from pregnancy-related causes and are suffering from severe health consequences like infertility. While other countries have reduced their infant mortality rates, the number of women who die from pregnancy-related causes in the U.S. has doubled in the last 25 years. And as we have heard this morning already, black women are three to four times more likely to die from pregnancy-related causes than white women, which is a truly shocking and appalling disparity.

Maternal mortality is also significantly higher in rural areas where obstetrical providers may not be available and delivery in rural hospitals is associated with higher rates of postpartum hemorrhage. March of Dimes will release a report in the coming weeks that will show that maternity care deserts exist in this country and in these deserts pregnant women face serious challenges in receiving appropriate care.

The state of maternal health in the United States is dire, but there are things we can do and we must do. Many factors are contributing to the maternal health crisis in this nation and our work to address it is important and it must be equally multifaceted. The bill before the subcommittee today is a critical step towards preventing death or serious health outcomes for pregnant women and new mothers.

The discussion draft of H.R. 1318, the Preventing Maternal Deaths Act, would provide grants to states and tribes to help establish or improve maternal mortality review committees or MMRCs. MMRCs are interdisciplinary groups of local experts that come together in maternal, infant, and public health to investigate the cases of maternal death, identify those system wide factors that contributed to these deaths, and then develop recommendations that would help prevent future cases.

MMRCs are unique in that they identify solutions. Not just collect the data, but then identify solutions that are targeted to the needs of pregnant women and mothers in specific states, cities, and communities. The discussion draft of H.R. 1318 would also establish a demonstration project to determine how best to address disparities in maternal health outcomes.

Mr. Chairman and members of the subcommittee, while this bill is extremely important, maternal mortality is not a single problem with a single solution. The causes of maternal mortality and severe maternal morbidity are diverse. They include physical health, mental health, social determinants, and much more. They can be traced back to the issues in our healthcare system including the quality of care as we just heard so passionately from Charles, systems problems, and of course the issue of implicit bias that exist in our healthcare system. They stem from factors in our homes, our workplaces, and our communities.

Mr. Chairman and members of the subcommittee, thank you for recognizing the urgency and the magnitude of this public health crisis. Our nation's mothers and babies cannot wait any longer. We must act now to save the lives and the health of pregnant women, new mothers, and their babies. Thank you.

[The prepared statement of Ms. Stewart follows:]

TESTIMONY OF STACEY D. STEWART, PRESIDENT, MARCH OF DIMES, BEFORE THE ENERGY AND COMMERCE SUBCOMMITTEE ON HEALTH, HEARING "BETTER DATA AND BETTER OUTCOMES: REDUCING MATERNAL MORTALITY IN THE U.S.," SEPTEMBER 27, 2018

Thank you, Mr. Chairman, for this opportunity to testify today before the Energy and Commerce Subcommittee on Health at this hearing, "Better Data and Better Outcomes: Reducing Maternal Mortality in the U.S." I am Stacey D. Stewart, President of March of Dimes, and I would like to commend you for holding this important hearing. March of Dimes is leading the fight for the health of all moms and babies.

Imagine, if you would, a classic hospital receiving blanket. It's made of soft white flannel, with a pastel blue and pink stripes on each end. Any of us with children will never forget that first moment when the doctor placed our precious baby boy or girl in our arms, wrapped warmly in one of these blankets. More than 700 times a year, a beautiful baby is wrapped up in a blanket just like this one - but there is no mother to hold that child. That is not just a statistic; 700 mothers die every year, and over 50,000 others experience dangerous complications that could have killed them — making the U.S. the most dangerous place in the developed world to give birth. This situation is completely unacceptable.

Our nation is in the midst of a crisis in maternal and child health. Across our nation, virtually every measure of the health of pregnant women, new mothers, and infants is going in the wrong direction. Preterm birth rates are rising. In many communities, infant mortality rates exceed those in developing nations. Nations like Slovenia and French Polynesia have a better infant mortality rate than the U.S.

Striking disparities exist among the health of mothers and babies of different racial and ethnic backgrounds. Black children face the highest child mortality rate among racial/ethnic groups – more than 2 times higher than the rate for Asian children and 1.5 times higher than the rate for white children.[1] There are dramatic variations in key measures like well-visits for women and infants among different racial and ethnic groups as well as geographic areas.

Maternal Mortality and Severe Maternal Morbidity Are a Public Health Crisis

Across the United States, women are tragically dying or suffering serious consequences from pregnancy-related causes. Despite the fact that many countries around the world have successfully reduced their maternal mortality rates since the 1990s, the U.S. rate is still higher than most other high-income countries,[2] and the U.S. maternal mortality rate has doubled in the past 25 years.[3] A significant racial and ethnic disparity in maternal mortality exists in the U.S., with black women being three to four times more likely to die from pregnancy-related causes compared to white women.[4,5]

Maternal mortality is also significantly higher in rural areas, where obstetrical providers may not be available,[6] and delivery in rural hospitals is associated with higher rates of postpartum hemorrhage.[7] March of Dimes will release a report in the coming weeks that will show these "maternity

---

[1] *America's Health Rankings Health of Women and Children Report.* March 2018. United Health Foundation. Available at https://assets.americashealthrankings.org/app/uploads/ahr_hwc_2018_report_summary_022818a.pdf.

[2] WHO. *Trends in Maternal Mortality 1990-2015.* Available at: http://www.who.int/reproductivehealth/publications/monitoring/maternal-mortality-2015/en/.

[3] CDC. Pregnancy Mortality Surveillance System. Available at: https://www.cdc.gov/reproductivehealth/maternalinfanthealth/pmss.html.

[4] Creanga AA, Berg CJ, Syverson C, Seed K, Bruce FC, Callaghan WM. Pregnancy-related mortality in the United States, 2006-2010. *Obstet Gynecol* 2015;125(1):5-12.

[5] Callaghan WM. Overview of maternal mortality in the United States. *Semin Perinatol* 2012;36(1):2-6.

[6] Faron, Dina. Maternal Health Care is disappearing in rural America. Scientific American, February 15, 2017.

[7] Kozhimannil KB, Thao V, Hung P, Tilden E, Caughey AB, Snowden JM. Association between hospital birth volume and maternal morbidity among low-risk pregnancies in rural, urban, and teaching hospitals in the United States. *Am J Perinatol* 2016 May;33(6):590-9.

care deserts," where pregnant women face serious challenges in receiving appropriate care.

Approximately 700 women die each year in the U.S. as a result of pregnancy or pregnancy-related complications.[8] The Centers for Disease Control and Prevention (CDC) estimates that up to 60% of these deaths are preventable.[9,10] For every maternal death, there are about 100 episodes of severe maternal morbidity (SMM) affecting more than 50,000 women in the United States every year.[11]

According to the CDC, pregnancy-related deaths are those that occur during pregnancy or within the following year due to pregnancy complications, because of a chain of events initiated by pregnancy, or because of an unrelated condition that was aggravated by pregnancy.[12] Severe maternal morbidity includes unexpected outcomes of labor and delivery that result in significant short or longer term consequences to a woman's health.[13]

Causes of maternal deaths include cardiovascular conditions, hypertensive disorders of pregnancy (preeclampsia/eclampsia), infection, hemorrhage, suicide and drug overdose. Identifying and treating medical conditions before, during and after pregnancy are essential to preventing maternal morbidity and maternal mortality, as part of the continuum of care for all women of childbearing age. This requires a commitment to high-quality clinical care and enhanced maternal quality improvement and safety initiatives in hospitals, particularly those that address disparities,

---

[8] MMRIA. *Report from Nine Maternal Mortality Review Committees*. February 2018. Available at: https://www.cdcfoundation.org/building-us-capacity-review-and-prevent-maternal-deaths.

[9] Berg CJ, Harper MA, Atkinson SM, et al. Preventability of pregnancy-related deaths: results of a state-wide review. *Obstet Gynecol* 2005;106(6):1228-1234.

[10] MMRIA. *Report from Nine Maternal Mortality Review Committees*. February 2018. Available at: https://www.cdcfoundation.org/building-us-capacity-review-and-prevent-maternal-deaths.

[11] CDC. *Severe Maternal Morbidity in the United States*. Available at: https://www.cdc.gov/reproductivehealth/maternalinfanthealth/severematernalmorbidity.html.

[12] CDC. *Pregnancy Mortality Surveillance System*. Available at: .https://www.cdc.gov/reproductivehealth/maternalinfanthealth/pmss.html.

[13] CDC. *Severe Maternal Morbidity in the United States*. Available at: https://www.cdc.gov/reproductivehealth/maternalinfanthealth/severematernalmorbidity.html.

structural barriers to care, differential care experienced by women of color, and provider implicit racial bias.[14]

March of Dimes supports efforts to eliminate preventable maternal mortality and SMM and the unacceptably large disparities in rates experienced by black women. To achieve this, March of Dimes:

- Encourages every state to have a maternal mortality review committee that investigates each death of a pregnant woman or new mother to understand causes and recommend interventions for the future.
- Supports efforts to improve ways to collect data on maternal mortality and SMM, research into their causes and prevention, and promotion of proven ways to keep all mothers healthy.
- Supports ensuring access to inpatient obstetrical facilities and qualified obstetrical providers in rural settings.
- Supports state perinatal quality collaboratives working with hospitals to identify and review cases of SMM and implement hospital based quality improvement initiatives to improve care and promote patient safety.
- Supports efforts to ensure that all women have quality, affordable health insurance and health care to include but not limited to postpartum depression screening, mental health treatment, substance use treatment, affordable contraception, including long-acting reversible contraception (LARC), and access to health care providers who understand and meet their health needs before, during and after pregnancy.
- Supports improving the social and economic conditions and quality of health care at all stages of a woman's life.
- Encourages acceleration of policies and programs shown to provide preventive and supportive care for women during pregnancy, including group prenatal care.

---

[14] Jain JA, Temming LA, D'Alton ME, et al. SMFM Special Report: Putting the "M" back in MFM: Reducing racial and ethnic disparities in maternal morbidity and mortality: A call to action. *Am J Obstet Gynecol* 2018;218(2):B9-B17.

The Preventing Maternal Deaths Act is a Critical Step Forward

The state of maternal health in the U.S. is dire, but there are things we can and must do. Many factors are contributing to the maternal health crisis in our nation, and our work to address it must be equally multi-faceted. The bill before the subcommittee today represents a critical step toward preventing death or serious health outcomes for pregnant women and new mothers.

The discussion draft of H.R. 1318, the Preventing Maternal Deaths Act, sponsored by Representatives Jaime Herrera Beutler (R-WA), Diana DeGette (D-CO) and Ryan Costello (R-PA) mirrors S. 1112, the Maternal Health Accountability Act, as recently passed by the Senate Committee on Health, Education, Labor and Pensions, would provide grants to states and tribes to help establish maternal mortality review committees (MMRCs) – interdisciplinary groups of local experts in maternal, infant and public health – to investigate cases of maternal death, identify system-wide factors that contributed to the deaths, and develop recommendations to prevent future cases. MMRCs are unique in that they identify solutions targeted to the needs of pregnant women and mothers in specific states, cities and communities. The discussion draft of H.R. 1318 would also establish a demonstration project to help ascertain how best to address disparities in maternal health outcomes. Together, these provisions will help us obtain the information and recommendations we need to prevent women from dying or experiencing serious health consequences of pregnancy. Congress should pass this important legislation as quickly as possible.

Our nation cannot prevent maternal mortality if we lack data about where and why it takes place. This legislation will fill significant gaps in our current knowledge by ensuring we have nationwide data on maternal mortality rates as well as information about causes. It will provide states and tribes with new resources to gather information and ensure their maternal mortality review committees operate according to best practices. Finally, it will protect the privacy of women and their families by ensuring strong confidentiality processes are in place to prevent the unauthorized release of information.

Mr. Chairman and members of the subcommittee, while this bill is extremely important, maternal mortality is not a single problem with a single solution. The causes of maternal mortality and severe maternal morbidity are diverse; they include physical health, mental health, social determinants, and much more. They can be traced back to issues in our health care system, including quality of care, systems problems, and implicit bias. They stem from factors in our homes, our workplaces, and our communities. The effort to save women's lives can't just end with one hearing and one bill. I urge Congress to launch a series of hearings into the root causes of maternal mortality and to pass additional measures to improve maternal and child health, because every mom and baby deserve a healthy start.

In conclusion, I would like to thank you, Mr. Chairman and members of the subcommittee, for recognizing the urgency and magnitude of this public health crisis. Our nation's mothers and babies cannot wait any longer. We must act now to save the lives and health of pregnant women, new mothers and their infants. Piecemeal efforts are not enough; moms and babies are dying. We need blanket change. March of Dimes stands ready to assist you in working to protect and improve the health of all women and babies.

Mr. BURGESS. Thank you, Ms. Stewart.

Dr. Coslett-Charlton, you are now recognized for 5 minutes, please.

STATEMENT OF LYNNE COSLETT-CHARLTON

Dr. COSLETT-CHARLTON. Chairman Burgess, Ranking Member Green, Chairman Walden, Ranking Member Pallone, and distinguished members of the Energy and Commerce Subcommittee on Health, thank you for inviting me to speak with you today on behalf of the American College of Obstetricians and Gynecologists at this hearing entitled, Better Data and Better Outcomes: Reducing Maternal Mortality in the U.S.

ACOG, with a membership of more than 58,000, is the leading physician organization dedicated to advancing women's health. Today's hearing will focus on a discussion draft of H.R. 1318, the Preventing Maternal Deaths Act, sponsored by Representatives Jaime Herrera Beutler, Diana DeGette, and Ryan Costello. I want to extend a special thank you to the bill sponsors for working so diligently on this bipartisan legislation, a critical first step in improving maternal health outcomes for women in this country.

A special thanks also to you, Dr. Burgess, my colleague OB/GYN, for your leadership highlighting this critically important issue and making maternal mortality a top priority.

As many of you know, the United States has a maternal mortality crisis. Too many women die each year in the United States from pregnancy-related and pregnancy-associated complications. We have higher maternal mortality rates than any other developed country. At a time when 157 of 183 countries in the world report decreases in maternal mortality, ours is rising. Black women are disproportionately affected and are three to four times more likely to lose their lives than white women. And for every maternal death in the United States there are a hundred women who experience severe maternal morbidity or near misses.

This is all unacceptable and the time for action is now. We know that over 60 percent of maternal deaths are preventable. Common causes include hemorrhage, cardiovascular and coronary conditions, cardiomyopathy, or infection. Overdose and suicide, driven primarily by the opioid epidemic, are also emerging as the leading causes of maternal mortality in a growing number of states including my own. If we have a clear understanding of why these deaths are occurring and what we can do to prevent them in the future, we can save women's lives.

The Preventing Maternal Death Act assists states in creating or expanding maternal mortality review committees through the Center of Disease Control and Prevention. MMRCs are multidisciplinary groups of local experts in maternal and public health as well as patient and community advocates that closely examine maternal death cases and identify locally relevant ways to prevent future deaths. While traditional public health surveillance using vital statistics can tell us about trends and disparities, MMRCs are the vehicle best positioned to comprehensively assess maternal deaths and identify, most importantly, opportunities for prevention.

As ACOG's Pennsylvania Section Chair and incoming District III Legislative Chair and a practicing physician for over 20 years, addressing maternal mortality is of critical importance to me. As an OB/GYN, seeing a woman die while pregnant or after delivering a baby is something that sticks with you for life and has stuck with me throughout my career. Preventing that kind of tragedy and ensuring the health and safety of the women we care for is central to our mission.

When I took over as ACOG's Pennsylvania Section Chair, Pennsylvania did not have MMRC, though the city of Philadelphia did. And over the past 2 ½ years I have worked diligently to organize the campaign with other OB/GYNs and other advocates in my state and the Department of Health to urge the state legislators to pass legislation to form our first statewide MMRC. Finally, on May 9th, Governor Wolf signed the Maternal Mortality Review Act. Our first meeting is next week. Enthusiasm like this for MMRCs is growing all over the country. Today, approximately 33 states have MMRC and as many of those 33, including Pennsylvania, are brand new this year.

But states like ours need help. The CDC plays a vital role in assisting these states to ensure their MMRCs are robust, multidisciplinary, and using standardized reporting, which is why it is important to have this federal legislation as mechanisms.

The Building U.S. Capacity to Prevent Maternal Deaths Initiative, a partnership between the CDC's National Center for Chronic Disease Prevention and Health Promotion, the CDC Foundation, the Association for Maternal & Child Health Programs, and Merck for Mothers has made tremendous progress giving technical assistance to states to help them establish MMRCs or ensure established MMRCs are operating with evidence-based practices.

In Pennsylvania we need to ensure that this type of technical assistance is amplified so that we can get our MMRC off the ground and working correctly. Once MMRCs are up and running they lead to opportunities for quality improvement. For example, to participate in the Alliance for Innovation on Maternal Health, or AIM, a state must first have an MMRC. AIM convened under ACOG's leadership is a national alliance of clinicians, hospital administration, patient safety organizations, and patient advocates that work to reduce maternal mortality and severe morbidity by creating condition-specific bundles which are evidence-based toolkits to improve maternal outcomes. Some of these bundles include severe hypertension, maternal mental health, obstetric care for women with opioid use disorder, obstetric hemorrhage, and racial disparities in maternity care. To participate in AIM, a state must first have MMRC. The data recommendations from MMRCs instruct states where they need to invest to address specific conditions that affect women in their community and ensure proper appropriate targeting of limited resources.

For us to clearly understand why women are dying from preventable maternal complications across the country and make lasting improvements, every state must have a robust MMRC. The Preventing Maternal Death Act will help us reach that goal and ultimately improve maternal health across this country. Thank you very much for the opportunity to speak to you about this pressing issue and in support of this very important legislation.

[The prepared statement of Dr. Coslett-Charlton follows:]

Written Testimony of the American College of Obstetricians and Gynecologists, Submitted by: Lynne Coslett-Charlton, MD, FACOG, before the House Energy and Commerce Subcommittee on Health, Regarding the Subcommittee Hearing, Better Data and Better Outcomes: Reducing Maternal Mortality in the U.S., September 27, 2018

Chairman Burgess, Ranking Member Green, Chairman Walden, Ranking Member Pallone, and distinguished Members of the Energy & Commerce Subcommittee on Health, thank you for inviting me to speak with you today on behalf of the American College of Obstetricians and Gynecologists (ACOG) at this hearing entitled, "Better Data and Better Outcomes: Reducing Maternal Mortality in the U.S." ACOG, with a membership of more than 58,000, is the leading physician organization dedicated to advancing women's health. Today's hearing will focus on a discussion draft of H.R. 1318, the Preventing Maternal Deaths Act, sponsored by Representatives Jaime Herrera Beutler, Diana DeGette, and Ryan Costello. I want to extend a special thank you to the bill sponsors for working so diligently on this bipartisan legislation – a critical first step in improving maternal health outcomes for women in this country. Special thanks also to you, Dr. Burgess, a colleague obgyn, for your leadership highlighting this critically important issue and making maternal mortality a top priority.

As many of you may know, the United States has a maternal mortality crisis. Too many women die each year in the United States from pregnancy-related or pregnancy-associated complications.[15] We have a higher maternal mortality rate than in any other developed country. At a

[15] Building U.S. Capacity to Review and Prevent Maternal Deaths. (2018). Report from nine maternal mortality review committees. Retrieved from http://reviewtoaction.org/Report_from_Nine_MMRCs.

time when 157 of 183 countries in the world report decreases in maternal mortality, ours is rising.[16] Black women are disproportionately affected and are three to four times more likely to lose their lives than white women.[17] For every maternal death in the United States, there are 100 women who experience severe maternal morbidity, or a "near miss." This is all unacceptable, and the time for action is now.

We know that over 60 percent of maternal deaths are preventable.[18] Common causes include hemorrhage, cardiovascular and coronary conditions, cardiomyopathy, or infection. Overdose and suicide, driven primarily by the opioid epidemic, are also emerging as the leading causes of maternal mortality in a growing number of states.[19] If we have a clear understanding of why these deaths are occurring, and what we can do to prevent them in the future, we can save women's lives.

The Preventing Maternal Deaths Act assists states in creating or expanding maternal mortality review committees (MMRCs) through the Centers for Disease Control and Prevention (CDC). MMRCs are multidisciplinary groups of local experts in maternal and public health, as well as patient and community advocates, that closely examine maternal death cases and identify locally-relevant ways to prevent future deaths. While traditional public health surveillance using vital statistics can tell us about trends and disparities, MMRCs are best positioned to comprehensively assess maternal deaths and identify opportunities for prevention.

As ACOG's Pennsylvania Section Chair, incoming ACOG District III Legislative Chair, and practicing physician for over 20 years, addressing maternal mortality is of critical importance to me. As an obgyn, seeing a woman die while pregnant or after delivering a baby is something that sticks with you for life. Preventing that kind of tragedy and ensuring the

---

[16] Lu MC. Reducing Maternal Mortality in the United States. *JAMA*. Published online September 10, 2018. doi:10.1001/jama.2018.11652.

[17] Pregnancy Mortality Surveillance System. Centers for Disease Control and Prevention. Available at: https://www.cdc.gov/reproductivehealth/maternalinfanthealth/pmss.html.

[18] *Building U.S. Capacity to Review and Prevent Maternal Deaths*. (2018). Report from nine maternal mortality review committees. Retrieved from http://reviewtoaction.org/Report_from_Nine_MMRCs.

[19] Ibid.

health and safety of the women we care for is central to our mission. When I took over as ACOG Pennsylvania Section Chair, Pennsylvania didn't have a maternal mortality review committee, though the city of Philadelphia did. Over the past two years, I have worked diligently to organize a campaign with other obgyns and advocates to urge the state legislature to pass legislation to form a statewide MMRC. Finally, on May 9, 2018, the governor signed the Maternal Mortality Review Act.

Enthusiasm like this for MMRCs is growing all over the country. Today, approximately 33 states have an MMRC – and many of those 33, including Pennsylvania, are brand new this year.[20] But states like ours need help. CDC plays a vital role in assisting these states to ensure their MMRCs are robust, multidisciplinary, and using standardized reporting mechanisms. The Building U.S. Capacity to Prevent Maternal Deaths initiative – a partnership between the CDC's National Center for Chronic Disease Prevention and Health Promotion, the CDC Foundation, the Association for Maternal & Child Health Programs, and Merck for Mothers – has made tremendous progress giving technical assistance to states to help them establish MMRCs or ensure established MMRCs are operating with evidence-based practices. In Pennsylvania, we need to ensure that this type of technical assistance is amplified, so we can get our MMRC off the ground and working correctly.

Once MMRCs are up and running, they lead to opportunities for quality improvement. For example, to participate in the Alliance for Innovation on Maternal Health, or AIM, a state must have an MMRC. AIM, convened under ACOG's leadership, is a national alliance of clinicians, hospital administrators, patient safety organizations, and patient advocates that work to reduce maternal mortality and severe maternal morbidity by creating condition-specific "bundles" – evidence-based toolkits to improve maternal outcomes. Some of these bundles include: severe hypertension, maternal mental health, obstetric care for women with opioid use disorder, obstetric hemorrhage, and racial disparities in maternity care.

---

[20] Ibid.

To participate in AIM, states must have an MMRC. The data and recommendations from MMRCs instruct states where they need to invest to address specific conditions that affect women in their community and ensure appropriate targeting of limited resources.

For us to clearly understand why women are dying from preventable maternal complications across the country and make lasting improvements, every state must have a robust MMRC. The Preventing Maternal Deaths Act will help us reach that goal, and ultimately improve maternal health across this country.

Thank you for the opportunity to speak to you about this pressing issue and in support of this important legislation. I'm happy to answer any questions.

Mr. BURGESS. Thank you, Dr. Charlton.

Dr. Crear Perry, you are recognized for 5 minutes, please.

STATEMENT OF JOIA CREAR PERRY

Dr. PERRY. So, thank you fellow ACOG member, Dr. Burgess. Mr. BURGESS. And if you will suspend for a moment, in the interest of full disclosure I am a dues-paying member of the American College of Obstetricians and Gynecologists.

Dr. PERRY. Here we go.

Mr. BURGESS. And I am current on that. And I don't do the emeritus stuff, I pay the full freight. You may proceed.

Dr. PERRY. And Ranking Member Green, thank you as well, and to my fellow colleagues on the panel. I really feel like going last is always a great way to go because you can hear what the gap might be in explaining this.

I get to work with the 33 states who are doing the MMRCs. As an organization we provide technical assistance. We also get to work in places like Philadelphia. We have been doing it for awhile. So a concrete example would be in Philadelphia they had a lot of women who were dying from cardiomyopathy, which sounds really medical, right, because your heart fails, it won't pump as well. When they actually reviewed the deaths, many of the women had heroin addiction, right, so it was something you could prevent if you actually put in mental healthcare services for addiction. So it is important for us to have a broader view.

Someone brought up California, which is really important. So California has decreased their deaths, but they still have a racial disparity. Still, in California despite having these great outcomes, they have had increased deaths for black women. So what they are doing now is really going back to look at implicit bias that was mentioned, making sure that their providers are culturally cognizant and having really some rules around what does it mean if you don't value a woman and she is not seen for several hours, how does that system respond to that and what can we do differently to ensure that people are seen in an appropriate amount of time.

So just wanted to give some teeth to how important this is and how having the ability to actually look at the deaths individually and to talk to family members and to have mental health there really can help us to get to some answers.

So now I want to tell you a little bit of my own story, because every woman's story needs to be heard and this is what the MMRC allows you to do. So when I was a third-year medical student in my home of Louisiana after attending Princeton for undergrad, my then-husband and I were expecting our planned second child. At about 5 ½ months pregnant, my water broke. My mother, who is here and a pharmacist, still recounts how panic-stricken she was when she was counseled by my physician about the risk of infection to my son and I that included death.

I had access to excellent health care for him provided by my health insurance coverage, but the stress of racism was my only risk factor for the premature birth of my son. The hospital where I was training was named Confederate Memorial just 20 years prior to this. Luckily, my 22-year-old son and I survived, but the sad reality is that my 25-year-old daughter has a higher risk of dying in childbirth than I did when I had her. The same is true for all of us who have daughters in the United States. We are failing our daughters, especially our black daughters who are dying at three to four times the rate of their white counterparts.

So, ultimately, what we are asking for this bill, when you think about what Charles said and what all of us have said, is we can no longer delay acting. This bill has been reiterated many times in Congress and I am excited to hear that maybe we can have it done by the end of this year, because it is important for us to say that we as a country—I got to testify at the U.N. about this very issue— the world is watching us. The world sees us. I get flown to Geneva to talk about how important it is for the United States to actually value women and to pay for and look at why women are dying, so this is an opportunity for us to say yes, we do value women and yes, we do want to see what is actually happening to them.

So ultimately what women, especially black women, in the United States need is accountability. We need to know that our lives are valued. We need to know that this accountability might be difficult, it might be complicated, but government still has an obligation to act. Accountability is a value that all Americans can agree upon, yet racism, classism, and gender oppression are killing all of us from rural to urban America. This is not about intentions. Lack of action is unintentionally killing us. It is a human rights imperative. We just ensure that prevention efforts and resources are being directed towards the areas of greatest need and be willing to name the problem directly.

Much can be accomplished through improving monitoring and data collection.

Me and my big writing because my eyes are getting bad, I am getting old.

H.R. 1318 is a tremendous step forward in showing that we do recognize, yes, black mamas matter. That is it.

[The prepared statement of Dr. Perry follows:]

September 25, 2018

Testimony of Joia Crear - Perry, MD, Founder and President, National Birth Equity Collaborative, Advisory Board Member, Black Mamas Matter Alliance, before the Subcommittee on Health Committee on Energy and Commerce, U.S. House of Representatives, "Better Data and Better Outcomes: Reducing Maternal Mortality the U.S.," 10:00 A.M., Friday, September 27, 2018

Good Morning Mr. Chairman, Ranking Member Green, members of the House Committee on Energy and Commerce Health Subcommittee for allowing me, Dr. Joia Crear-Perry, to testify at this Better Data and Better Outcomes: Reducing Maternal Mortality in the US hearing representing the National Birth Equity Collaborative and the Black Mamas Matter Alliance.

H.R.1318 will support states in their work to save and sustain the health of mothers during pregnancy, childbirth, and in the postpartum period. Of vital importance to my reproductive justice peers and I, it will work to eliminate disparities across maternal health outcomes for pregnancy-related and pregnancy-associated deaths. H.R. 1318, working with groups such as ours, will also identify solutions to improve health care quality and health outcomes for mothers.

As you may be aware, the United States is the only developed country in the world where maternal mortality is on the rise. Further, Black women in the U.S. die at 3 to 4 times the rate of their white counterparts. Despite clear evidence of this inequity, policymakers, and as a consequence, government had not, until now, addressed this urgent public health and human rights issue. The Centers for Disease Control defines Pregnancy Related death as the death of a woman while pregnant or within one year of the end of a pregnancy – regardless of outcome, duration or site of the pregnancy – from any cause related to or aggravated by pregnancy or its management. Based on that definition, the CDC found in their surveillance, 2,726 women died in the United States between 2011 and 2014 and of those 1,010 or 38% were Black. As a Black woman from the Deep South, who is an obstetrician and a mother, my strong desire to end this inequity is amplified every time I look into the faces of my daughter and patients.

As a Black mother, I cannot buy or educate my way out of dying at 3 to 4 times the rate of a white mother in the United States. The inequity in maternal mortality rates persists regardless of our income or education status. A White woman with less than a high school education has a better chance to live in childbirth than a Black woman with a college degree. The legacy of a hierarchy of human value based on the color of our skin continues to cause differences in health outcomes, including maternal mortality. Racism is the risk factor – not Black skin. There is no "Black" gene.

Maternal mortality extends beyond the period of pregnancy or birth. Nine months of prenatal care cannot counter underlying social determinants of health inequities in housing, political participation, transportation, education, food, environmental conditions, and economic security; all of which have racism as their root cause. We have data that shows that a Black woman who initiates prenatal care in the first trimester has a worse outcome in birth than a white woman with late or no prenatal care.

Good maternal health outcomes depend upon implementation of all sexual and reproductive rights, from comprehensive sexual education to access to all forms of birth control. We know that Medicaid Expansion is critical to ensuring that Maternal Mortality rates improve across our great nation. We have data that shows that this investment in states, such as my own great state of Louisiana, saves money and lives. Even if women are insured, coverage of sexual and reproductive health services is too often not comprehensive. Receiving the full range of reproductive options ensures safe healthy births for moms and babies. Reproductive life planning in schools, health facilities, community organizations and homes, reinforces the tools our future generations need to make healthy choices about when, how and if, they want to have children to optimize their physical, emotional and fiscal health in order to build a stronger, more secure nation.

Closures of hospitals and maternity units create barriers to services and information. This lack of a safety net for poor and rural Americans produces gaps in access along the reproductive life span. This includes closures of rural hospitals from Texas, Kentucky, Michigan, Illinois, Tennessee, Ohio, Washington, New Jersey, Virginia, Florida, Missouri, Indiana, Oklahoma, North Carolina, Georgia, Oregon, New York, California, Maryland, New Mexico, Massachusetts, and Colorado. All of us are impacted when we make choices to defund Critical Access facilities and disinvest in communities that we deem not economically viable. As someone who grew up in rural America, I watched my best friend have her baby in the car on the way to the hospital that was an hour away. That child has severe cerebral palsy. What is the value of these often forgotten communities and families? What are we saying about how we value them in our policy and funding priorities?

I am the founder of the National Birth Equity Collaborative and on the Advisory Committee for the Black Mamas Matter Alliance. The National Birth Equity Collaborative envisions a world where every Black baby lives to their first birthday with their family. The Black Mamas Matter Alliance serves as a national voice and coordinating entity for stakeholders advancing maternal health, rights, and justice, and intentionally centers Black women's leadership. BMMA has a network of organizations with the reach, relationships and capacity to support an intergenerational movement. BMMA organizes around four core strategies which aim to 1) advance policy that addresses black maternal health inequity 2) cultivate innovative research methods, 3) enhance holistic and comprehensive approaches to the care of black mamas, and 4) shift culture of the narratives of black motherhood by amplifying black women's voices.

The Maternal Mortality Review is a process by which a multidisciplinary committee at the state or local jurisdiction level identifies and reviews cases of maternal death within one year of pregnancy. Review Committees often include representatives from the areas of public health, obstetrics and gynecology, maternal-fetal medicine, nursing, midwifery, forensic pathology, mental health and behavioral health. Review Committees have access to multiple sources of information that provide a deeper understanding of the circumstances surrounding the death and develop action recommendations to prevent future deaths. According to the CDC, currently at least 36 states and 3 Cities have or are forming a Maternal Mortality Review Committee. Very few are fully functioning due to lack of fiscal support.

Data availability and transparency is important. While making the reports available to the Centers for Disease Control ensures data quality and that we are able to look at national trends in maternal mortality and morbidity, state and local level entities and advocacy organizations also need access to data and reports to inform maternal health programs and services. Additionally, timely availability of reports equips these advocates with critical information to influence policy decisions that are impacting their communities directly.

I applaud the expanded focus of the bill to include severe maternal morbidity. While maternal mortality in the U.S. is on the rise, data reflects that severe maternal morbidity is 100 times more common, impacting even more women and families. To acknowledge women experiencing a severe maternal morbidity is to recognize that there are women suffering, at times, life-long consequences and medical complications as a result of pregnancy and childbirth.

I also applaud the bill's recognition of the value of community engagement and inclusion in the maternal mortality review process. Mandating that by a state's participation in the program, the maternal mortality review committee shall include "individuals and organizations that represent the populations ...most affected by pregnancy-related deaths or pregnancy-associated deaths and lack of access to maternal health care services" is critical. We must hold states accountable to this mandate. The individuals and communities impacted by this issue must have a seat at the table when discussing programs and policies that directly impact their health and access to health care services.

Ultimately, what Black women in the U.S. need is accountability. We need to know that our lives are valued. This accountability may be complicated, but government still has an obligation to act. Racism, classism and gender oppression are killing all of us, from rural to urban America. This is not about intentions. Lack of action is "unintentionally" killing us. It is a human rights imperative. Throughout the bill, there is no mention of race, racism, or racial disparities. The inability to name this as a key focus to reduce RACIAL disparities in maternal mortality and morbidity will continue to exacerbate the problem. We must ensure that prevention efforts and resources are being directed toward the areas of greatest need and be willing to name the problem directly.

Much can be accomplished through improved monitoring and data collection. H.R.1318 is a tremendous step forward in showing that we do recognize…Yes, Black Mamas Matter.

Mr. BURGESS. Thank you, Dr. Perry, Dr. Crear Perry. I appreciate your testimony and appreciate all of our witnesses for being here.

I will move to the question part of the hearing and I will recognize myself 5 minutes for questions. And Dr. Coslett-Charlton, let me ask you as a—we have heard the stories and yes, the review committees are important, legislation is important. But honestly, doctor to doctor, it is decisions that are made at the bedside and I honestly don't know how you legislate correct decisions to be made at the bedside.

So as part of this effort and as a fellow member in the American College of OB/GYN, it is really incumbent upon our professional societies, medical societies, our specialty society. This is where the rubber meets the road. We have to be—I don't know how I can legislate something that stops what Mr. Johnson went through. I just don't know how I can do that. Here was a situation where all the signs and symptoms pointed to exsanguination and he describes unfortunately in very painful detail what the natural consequence of exsanguination is, and I don't know how I write legislation to stop that from happening. That is on us as a profession, right?

Dr. COSLETT-CHARLTON. I totally agree. And I think that is why we are here and that is why we are sitting beside Mr. Johnson because those stories, I think, affect. And I know, Dr. Burgess, because you practiced for so long, I look at my intern year, I was on my internal medicine critical care rotation, probably the second month of rotation and I was called for a code for one who had a very rare condition called an amniotic fluid embolism, which I don't know if you have seen one in your career, but I was like what could this be—one in 300,000—and she died in front of me.

I was an intern observing, I wasn't actively participating in the care at that time, but I seriously questioned whether or not I wanted to go into this field at that time because—and I am so glad I did, because the joy of being an OB/GYN far outweighs the unfortunate things that happen to patients sometimes. But I think seeing that, if we can prevent one death, if we can educate our members, and really the best way to do that is to understand where the problems lie.

And the AIM programs are a great success story and if we are able to roll them out across the country and really see where we can use best practices to prevent things from happening that couldn't otherwise, and really obstetric hemorrhage is a perfect example where having the beauty of the AIM program is that it is, really, readiness first, so the four Rs, readiness and then recognize that there is a problem. So the readiness includes things like having suture available, having medication available on the labor floor so that you are not calling a pharmacist to come, I need this medicine now not an hour from now while you approve it.

So being ready, being able to recognize that there is a problem and educating staff members. Not just physicians, but also people that are on the front lines caring for the patients first. And also the response and having protocols for response that are appropriate, having blood products readily available for women when they are in transfusion protocols we have shown to be effective.

And, finally, reporting, because when we talk about maternal mortality and we talk about the deaths that is very important, but also the near misses are equally devastating and equally important that we know how to identify them. And not only, we are seeing the iceberg, if we can really get to the crux of that where we are truly going to improve the way we care for women in this country and I am positive we are going to see fewer maternal deaths.

Mr. BURGESS. Well, and that is what is critical about this. Maternal mortality review committees, I think that is an excellent idea. I am all in favor of that. I will just say in the 1970s at Parkland Hospital it was called grand rounds. And you didn't ever want to present at grand rounds. That probably meant your patient hadn't done well, but what it really meant was you weren't going to do well for the next couple of hours. And Dr. Jack Pritchard was the head of the department back then. He was pretty critical and had a way of asking those insightful questions that exposed any perhaps weakness in your clinical judgment or your thought process as you worked through a complicated issue.

Let me just ask you, have we gotten away as a profession from that type of introspection that you probably were exposed to in residency? I know I was.

Dr. COSLETT-CHARLTON. No, I think if you speak to any residents those processes still happen, but they happen mainly in academic centers. And really a part of this problem is that we have to better reach the communities. I practice in a small community hospital right now and it is very different. I think and educating practitioners in the community hospitals we know is equally as important, and access to care obviously as we have spoken to is equally important.

So I think being able to collect the data, being able to see where the deficiencies and having a mechanism and a vehicle and support nationally down to the state levels and the tentacles that can get the boots on the ground to make sure that none of these things happen anywhere in the United States is critical.

Mr. BURGESS. Well, Mr. Green gets extremely critical of me if I run over, so I will yield back my time and recognize the gentleman from Texas for 5 minutes for questions.

Mr. GREEN. I just ask equal time, Mr. Chair. I want to thank all our witnesses. And, Mr. Johnson, being a father of two children and now a grandfather, I just, and as the chair said, I don't think there is anything we can do. Of course there is no shortage. We have a lot of doctors in Congress but we also have a lot of lawyers. And so people say well, you can go to the tort system, and but that is not going to bring back your wife or your second baby. And it just, how do you do that? But we understand, those of us who have children and I know physicians particularly.

So I want to thank all of our witnesses today being here and discussing the U.S.'s maternal mortality rate, which I would be remiss if I didn't acknowledge my home state's maternal mortality crisis as well. As widely reported in 2016, published in Obstetrics & Gynecology found the Texas maternal rate was doubled between 2010 and 2012. The study's authors acknowledge these statistics were unexplainably high.

In the wake of this chapter, Texas' Maternal Mortality and Morbidity Task Force underwent review of all pregnancy-related deaths in Texas to determine the accuracy of these findings. What the task force found was that data collection errors and lack of standardization in reporting has resulted in varying statistics. If we can't depend on the research, that is a problem.

Dr. Coslett-Charlton, can you explain why the standardization of data collection is so critical when discussing maternal death rates?

Dr. COSLETT-CHARLTON. That is a very important question, Representative Green. And I think the crux of the issue is that the vehicles of looking at vital statistic records we are able in the pregnancy checkboxes, if someone pregnant within a year or 42 days in Texas of delivery that those measures certainly can identify and are inherent to error.

But the important thing and why we are here today is to make sure that all of those deaths are reviewed so that we can have accurate data. And that is why these maternal mortality review committees are essential, because not only are they going to review the deaths but they are going to be able to determine if they could have been preventable deaths and that is where the impact truly could be made.

Mr. GREEN. What can we learn from this study in Texas, and tell me Texas is not the only state that has that kind of statistics that you can't depend on. Is it other states, in Pennsylvania, or other states in the country?

Dr. COSLETT-CHARLTON. Well, in Pennsylvania we have had the checkbox for the past 5 years and I think that in Philadelphia there has been a small community that they have been able to focus on that data. But

I think like I was saying, the essential part of this is that having accurate data is really, really, truly important and the Texas studies truly exemplify that how important these MMRCs are.

The Texas committee at that time was not as sophisticated as it is now and their means of collecting aren't as sophisticated, so I think that going forward it is a perfect example of why this is essential.

Mr. GREEN. The Texas Maternal Mortality and Morbidity Task Force put out a series of recommendations on ways to improve maternal health and prevent pregnancy-related complications. Just this last month, the task force released its joint biannual report for our Department of State Health Services. Their first recommendation is we increase access to healthcare services to improve the health of women, facilitate continuity of care, and enable an effective care transitions and promote safe birth spacing.

Dr. Crear Perry, would you agree with the recommendation to improve maternal health we must improve the access to care?

Dr. PERRY. Sure. And I want to also piggyback on the last question a little bit about the data because it is important that we— it is a common phenomenon across the country, so it is not just Texas and it is not just Pennsylvania. A lot of states need this money to help with collect more accurate data, it would be really helpful.

And as far as access it is a big barrier. We see that places where closing rural hospitals in Texas, in Georgia, that when women have to travel an hour to have a baby they are more likely to hemorrhage. They are more likely to have a heart attack. They are more likely to have these medical conditions. So if you don't have a systemic review you can't look at the match between where your access is being denied and where women are also dying in the same place. So having a more robust review of the deaths will allow you to look at that.

Mr. GREEN. From my perspective coming from Texas, one way to improve access to care is expanding access to Medicaid and ensuring low-income individuals have the care that they need. And do you agree with that?

Dr. PERRY. Sure. I am from the great State of Louisiana and so we have seen actual data since Louisiana expanded Medicaid. We are one of the few deep southern states that expanded Medicaid where we have had improved outcomes. Our governor, really it was important for him to ensure that we had access to Medicaid expansion. Women are getting preventive services so you know that you have diabetes before you become pregnant and you don't show up at the hospital pregnant with uncontrolled blood sugars. So it is important that we have expanded Medicaid.

Mr. GREEN. And in my last 9 seconds, there is no replacement for prenatal care and having a mother who has a relationship with their doctor and that is why we need to have that access no matter who pays for it—Medicare, private sector or whatever.

So, Mr. Chairman, thank you for your time.

Mr. BURGESS. The chair thanks the gentleman. The gentleman yields back. The chair recognizes the gentleman from Kentucky, Mr. Guthrie, the vice chair of the committee, 5 minutes for questions.

Mr. GUTHRIE. Thank you, Mr. Chairman, and I appreciate everybody being here.

Mr. Johnson, I appreciate you coming here and being willing to share your story. I know that a lot of times we have policy developed and things develop because people went through tragic things and they are willing to bring that to our attention and share. And I know it is difficult to do, but it is one way that they live on and it is a way that it actually changes what is going on in the country, so we appreciate that.

And this is something that has been on the mind of the committee, I know the chairman, I know from his background, but also I remember being in a meeting earlier and we were trying to just get down to the policy that needs to happen. And your story, I remember one of the roundtables that the chairman has talking about the—it is not just access to care. It sounds like your wife was in a fantastic hospital situation and everything and it seems C-sections were something that could be common.

And we are the most, it is not that people aren't getting care. A lot of people are getting C-sections. And my wife has had—I have three children, we have had three, so it really made me cringe when I heard that in your story, because it seems the second or third or whatever, C-sections seem to be something that is something we need to address in moving forward and that gets to just finding the right data.

And Dr. Coslett-Charlton—Charlton or Charlton? Charlton. I know you are with ACOG and in this bill today we are looking at data and how to move data. I know ACOG has endorsed—a number of medical societies and ACOG has endorsed this bill and it is my hope that we can get sound data to see exactly the actions that we need to take. So can you speak to ACOG's perspective on the role of data in your efforts to reduce maternal mortality?

Dr. COSLETT-CHARLTON. So I think to some degree when you are speaking about specific situations like C-section rates and talking about, you know, once a woman has a first C-section, second C-section, third C-section, we know each time that a woman has a C-section risk can increase with subsequent pregnancies. And those are important reasons why, number one, we need access to good care.

But also, the part of the AIM bundles where we talk about preparedness or readiness is that when we know a woman has a third C-section, knowing that you could—if she has the ability to have important prenatal care to recognize the potential complications and be ready for those complications, that is critical and essential.

And the last thing, if we talk about the AIM bundles, one of the bundles is looking at how to improve primary Caesarean section rates so that is something that is good data that is coming out of California that we hope can translate, sharing data across state lines. Women are women in Pennsylvania the same as in Arizona. So, it really isn't rocket science. We should be able to share data and establish best practices and the way to do that is to have the vehicle or the mechanism to accurately be able to identify and look through that data.

Mr. GUTHRIE. It just seems standard—not being a physician at all, I am a manufacturing person—but it just seems to be standard now that if somebody is having their second or third C-section that the symptoms your wife showed seems to be clear from what you said that maybe there should be a team waiting to see if something happens and being ready for any type of those. I would love if you wanted to comment.

Mr. JOHNSON. Absolutely. I think that the astronomical C-section rates are something that needs to be examined. When we talk about Kira's case, there was a C-section, indeed, but it wasn't the C-section that led to her ultimate passing. And I will share this with the committee and I didn't share—what I had shared earlier was a very condensed version of what was happening to Kira.

But what we found subsequently when we go back and look at the medical records, which I shared as part of my record, is that in Kira's case she was exceptionally healthy, she went in for a routine scheduled C-section. And from what I understand, and Dr. Burgess and some of the medical people here, is what I understand is that for a woman who is having a Caesarean section, the cut timing and the time that they make the incision until the time that the baby is born, for a healthy woman and the baby is not under stress should be between 12 and 15 minutes. Is that fair, Dr. Burgess? OK. And in a situation where a woman has had a previous Caesarean you should add another 3 to 5 minutes so that you can cut around the scar tissue.

Mr. GUTHRIE. The problems with scar tissue in the second or third, Dr. Burgess explained that to me.

Mr. JOHNSON. Yes. So this is the point I would like to make is, so we are talking about between 15 to 20 minutes, ballpark, for a woman that is healthy, second Caesarean section, the baby is not in distress. When we received the medical records from Cedars-Sinai Hospital, the cut time on the delivery for my second son, Langston, was less than 2 minutes. Less than 2 minutes. And in the process of him rushing he lacerated her bladder.

But once again, and so the way that has been described is that this was not a medical tragedy, this was a medical catastrophe meaning that everything that could have gone wrong did go wrong.

So let's talk a minute about AIM which is a phenomenal program. And I want to salute ACOG for the work that they are doing in conjunction with AIM and being rolled out in various states. California, where we were where my son was delivered, is one of the trademark states for AIM and what they have done to reduce the maternal mortality rate with their hemorrhage bundle. But as long as we have these tools that are a suggestion and they are not a protocol, women are going to continue to pass away.

So the AIM bundle was available in Kira's case. It is one of the— it is ground zero for the wonderful work they have done reducing the maternal mortality rate in California, but they just chose to ignore it and I continued to beg and plead while her condition deteriorated.

So Caesareans are a challenge, but in Kira's——

Mr. GUTHRIE. Different.

Mr. JOHNSON. She was extremely healthy and they just let her continue to deteriorate. So we have got to have a fundamental standard of care that is not just a suggestion as AIM, as it is in the situation with AIM—and it is phenomenal—but if we can make a fundamental standard of care across the board that will make a big difference.

Mr. GUTHRIE. Thank you. Thank you for sharing and my time has expired. I yield back.

Mr. BURGESS. Thank you, Mr. Guthrie.

Mr. Ca´rdenas, you are recognized for 5 minutes, please, for questions.

Mr. CA´RDENAS. Thank you very much. And to Mr. Johnson, it is just amazing and incredible that you are doing what you are doing and thank you so much. You are saving lives and I appreciate that very much and so does everybody in this country and the world who will benefit from hopefully good decisions that we make, all of your efforts.

First, I would like to ask some questions if the doctors would— I recently read about a program in California that has been very successful since both the March of Dimes and the College of Obstetricians and Gynecologists are part of the California Maternal Quality Care Collaborative. I am hoping that both Dr. Coslett-Charlton and Ms. Stewart can tell us more about this program.

But in California's private-public partnership it was stressed that it was because of the views from a diverse panel of experts that they could avoid missing important details on women's deaths. And one of the things that I think it is important for us to understand is—I have been given a chart about the red line shows the mortality rate across the country while the highlighted yellow line actually shows California's. And we see a dramatic drop since 2007 when California has implemented the process of teaching each other, learning from each other, sharing data. And you are looking at California that has a mortality rate of 7.3 per 100,000 and across the country it is still up at 22.

So what I would like to see happen is we as Congress and those of us who are involved, or those of you who are involved on the day-to-day process that we can come together and create a national best practices, and I hope that that is the outcome not only at this hearing but of this Congress.

Dr. Coslett-Charlton and Ms. Stewart, if you can, can you talk a bit about how the diversity of these panels has changed and improved the maternal outcomes?

Ms. STEWART. Well, let me just start with a couple of points, which is I think that it is notable that California has had so much success, obviously, and I think the idea of the committee that has been formed, the way they have come together to look at data, to design interventions, identify where the problems are within the state and really design interventions that have made a meaningful difference has been important. And that is important to say at a high level, but again when it comes down to each individual person who still may be affected by the gaps in the system like Charles and like his wife Kira, then we still have a problem.

I want to say one thing about diversity in general and the importance of how this issue shows up and the disparate outcomes that many women of color experience as a result of the gaps in the system. And I agree with the chairman we can't legislate morality, but what we can do is ensure that we are tracking the performance of the system, we are tracking those women that are impacted disproportionately by the system, and that we are intentional in designing interventions that will make a difference.

The gaps in the system don't just start though when women show up in the hospital. They start well before then. We know that for example to make sure that we have healthier babies it doesn't just happen in the 9 months of pregnancy. And I am not a physician. I am not an OB/GYN, but I think I have known that in my own experience having had two babies and leading the March of Dimes, which is the leading organization in the fight for the health of moms and babies.

The same is true for healthier mothers. We have got to make sure that women have access to health care before they are pregnant especially if they have chronic diseases, chronic health challenges that might risk their health or the health of their baby. We have got to make sure they have access to good affordable care during pregnancy and what we know now is that it is important that women have access to excellent care after.

And it is especially important and we have had research and studies to show that women of color also feel less trust and less well-served by the system. They feel less listened to and respected in terms of their symptoms when they articulate those symptoms. And these are women that are not only low-income women of color, these are women that are affluent women of color, women that are highly educated who simply have reported—and again studies show this—that their needs are not being met at the same level at the same rate as white women and other women.

So I just want to say that I think this issue of diversity is really important not just in the panels but across the board in listening to the issues of disparate outcomes that we see across all communities.

Mr. CA´RDENAS. So best practices are something that we can improve and hopefully will become more prolific so we can have the outcomes that you just described. My time is limited, but hopefully during the testimony some of you can talk about the toolkits and how these toolkits are free.

But a quick, quick question to Mr. Johnson is since you have lost Kira, it has been 2 years, how has this affected you and your family, if you could describe that for us, so we can understand the true responsibility that we have and we can make sure that this happens less and less and less. Thank you.

Mr. JOHNSON. Well, this has been the most challenging experience that I could ever—even more challenging than anything that I could ever comprehend. That being said, the true blessing in all of this is the two tremendous gifts that Kira left us and that is my son Charles and my son Langston. They really, truly are what keeps myself, my mother who is seated behind me, all of us going.

And, it is difficult as they mature and as they are, now 2 and just turned 4 years old, their ability to process and understand the absence of their mother evolves. And like I said, when you talk to a 2 year old he wants to know why his mommy is not coming home. And you explain to him, well, your mother is in heaven and she is doing important work with God. And he tells you, well, I want to go to heaven too.

And so there is nothing that I can prepare for, there is nothing that I can do to fix that and I hope that over time that—the heart is saying to just be completely honest with you is I am proud to be here representing these families, but at the end of the day I am just a father that whose heart aches for his sons and a husband that misses his wife desperately. And so while there is every day I search for answers and how to support these amazing gifts, what I am clear about is that what I have to do is, although there is nothing I can do to bring Kira back I have to do everything that I can whenever I can to make sure that I send other mothers home with their babies.

And that if I can prevent another father from going through this, if I can prevent another child from having to understand why his mother isn't showing up at school—and I will share this with the committee. This is something that I have never even shared with my family, is when a 3-year-old asks you, Daddy, is Mommy mad at me? I want Mommy to come home. Why won't she come home? And I have never shared that with anybody because it is just too painful for me to articulate.

But I am clear that the work that we are doing here is going to prevent this to continue to happen to other women and it is going to make sure that other women get to go home with their babies.

Mr. CA´RDENAS. Mr. Chairman, if you will allow me a few seconds to thank Mr. Johnson, my time has expired. Thank you so much.

Thank you for your courage, your strength, and your commitment to community and to others and God bless you and your family. And know that your wife is doing good work in heaven, but you are doing tremendous work on earth. Thank you. I yield back.

Mr. BURGESS. The chair thanks the gentleman. The gentleman from California referenced the California Toolkit to Transform Maternity Care. I did print off a copy of that and at the conclusion of the hearing I will ask unanimous consent to make that as part of the record.

The chair now recognizes the gentleman from Ohio, Mr. Latta, 5 minutes for your questions, please.

Mr. LATTA. Thank you very much, Mr. Chairman. And thanks so much for our panel of witnesses and for being with us today because it is so important for the work that you are doing in getting this message out.

Ms. Stewart, if I could start my questioning, I am also concerned for soon-to-be mothers and new moms that live in our rural areas of our country. The national data indicates that more than half of all rural U.S. counties are without hospital obstetric services. With an increase of women dying due to pregnancy-related complications, how does access to care and hospital services affect pregnancies and postpartum recovery and is this issue exacerbated for women in our rural communities?

Ms. STEWART. Thank you very much. It is a very serious issue and thank you for the question. And as I mentioned in my statement earlier, the March of Dimes is working currently on a report that would really show this issue of maternity care deserts. The issue of the closing of community hospitals in rural areas has been well documented.

One of the things that we are missing is that it is not just the closing of hospitals. It is the closing of hospitals compounded by the lack of obstetrical services and OB/GYNs, the lack of midwives and doulas in areas, the distance that women often have to travel just to receive care, and it is particularly acute not just—in rural areas there is a major challenge, but one of the things we are looking at is even where in urban areas there can be maternity care deserts as well.

I will give you a good example of this. Here in the District of Columbia there is no hospital that provides obstetrical services east of the river in Wards 7 and 8. So east of the Anacostia River, tens of thousands of women who live there who have no hospital to go to, who then have to travel. If they have no transportation they have to go on the Metro often an hour or more to even go to a prenatal visit. If you are a high-risk pregnancy or you have a high-risk pregnancy, the complications that are then exacerbated or the complications that can result because of that distance, because that lack of access is increased significantly.

So one of the things that we really need to talk about in the system is the fact that even in the District of Columbia, for example, where there may be the number of beds may be sufficient for the number of women, that doesn't mean that those beds or that care is available to all the women that need it when they need it, and that is a very significant problem.

So I think one of the things that we are doing in the March of Dimes is to try to work with our friends in health care, our partners—ACOG has been a longtime partner of ours—working with hospitals and others to make sure that services are available.

The last thing I will just mention is that because all these issues that we are talking about today really just disproportionately again impact women of color. Women of color, African American women, are three to four times more likely to die as a result of childbirth. We also need to look at other ways in which services can be provided. We know that African American women, for example, are far more likely to want to receive services and care from a doula working within the formal healthcare system. And we have got to make sure that those services are also available so that women have places they can go they can trust. They know they go to places that will listen to them and that will respond to their needs and that will deal with their situation if they have high-risk needs as well. And what we are seeing today is that there are significant gaps in rural areas as well as in urban areas too.

Mr. LATTA. Dr. Coslett-Charlton, our country is facing an opioid epidemic and especially in the State of Ohio we are, unfortunately, about the third worst in the country. And while Congress and especially this committee has done a lot of work and we have passed a lot of bills trying to reverse this devastation, I can't help but think of the pregnant women and the new mothers who struggle with addiction.

And how prevalent is opioid abuse in maternal deaths?

Dr. COSLETT-CHARLTON. Well, I would comment that it is very significant and that is why it is so important that these maternal mortality review committees include diverse members including mental health professionals, substance abuse professionals and I know when we established our panel in Pennsylvania it was imperative that we had representatives from communities where—because that is a very significant issue and I know Philadelphia has seen a large increase. That they have done a good job of looking at their data, almost a doubling of maternal deaths over a short period of time related directly to the opioid abuse process.

And ACOG really appreciates all of the work that government is doing to make sure that—pregnant women are a special population that sometimes have different needs, so the pregnant addicted mother, number one, it is a great population to invest in because women that are pregnant that have opioid use disorders are often motivated to get better. You have a reason to get better. Not that everybody doesn't, but a pregnant woman is a special population.

And the other thing that we have seen is that doing, not only paying attention to different prescribing needs as we are limiting prescriptions, I see in my state things like that to make the special considerations for pregnant women that may have difficulties with access and need and to make sure that they continue on treatment during pregnancy and postpartum.

The last thing is that there are special pilot projects that are coming out of these committees looking at the special population of pregnant women, and like soft landing centers where we are not separating moms and babies, and, very importantly, not making punitive decisions based on maternal care and that because we know that women, the fear of losing their child or going into a system are not going to seek prenatal care and how imperative that is for the health of the woman and the child that she is carrying. So those are all things that ACOG is working very passionately on to try to improve the health care of women related to opioid use disorder.

Mr. LATTA. Well, thank you very much. And, Mr. Chairman, my time has expired and I yield back.

Mr. BURGESS. The chair thanks the gentleman. The gentleman yields back. The chair recognizes the gentlelady from Colorado, Ms. DeGette, 5 minutes for questions, please.

Ms. DEGETTE. Thank you so much, Mr. Chairman, and I want to thank all of our witnesses, but especially you, Mr. Johnson. I just can't even imagine what it must be like raising those two boys and I am glad your mom is here to help you. But, I want to come over and help myself, but I am not sure what I—and I think probably most of us feel that way if there is anything we can do.

I think the first thing we can do is pass this bill. And I have been working with my co-sponsor, Representative Herrera Beutler, to try to get this bill passed by the end of the year and I think your testimony is what will bring us over the line. So if people wonder, does it make a difference that answer would be yes, so thank you.

I want to ask you—am I pronouncing it correctly, Crear Perry? Crear Perry, OK. I want to ask you, Doctor, according to the CDC, the Nation's maternal mortality rate rose by 26 percent between 2000 and 2014; is that correct?

Dr. PERRY. Yes.

Ms. DEGETTE. One of the most striking aspects that I have been researching of this uptake is that African American women are nearly four times as likely to experience a pregnancy-related death than other women; is that right?

Dr. PERRY. It is. In some places it is higher.

Ms. DEGETTE. It is higher in some places?

Dr. PERRY. Yes. In New York City it was 12 to 1.

Ms. DEGETTE. Wow. And can you explain to me why this is? But it goes across——

Dr. PERRY. It does.

Ms. DEGETTE [continuing]. Socioeconomic lines, which is stunning. Can you explain a little bit about that for me?

Dr. PERRY. Well, and I think, for me, Charles' story really reflects this idea, right.

Ms. DEGETTE. Yes.

Dr. PERRY. Like in general in the United States we have not really grasped the idea that women, when they are pregnant, are special populations and it is important that we value them. So to have someone in the hospital for a long time without evaluating them, it means there is a fundamental lack of valuing them as a person and wanting to come and check on them. And saying she is not a priority right now and what we don't do when we just look individually at the doctor, it wasn't just the doctor. So a lawsuit, when you have an entire system and a structure——

Ms. DEGETTE. Just the whole hospital.

Dr. PERRY. And it is the whole structure. So how do we get to a space where black women and women in general, right? Because the reason that the gap is high in New York and not in Texas is because white women in Texas are dying. So it is not so much that black women are doing so great in Texas, so in general across this country.

Ms. DEGETTE. There is just fewer of them.

Dr. PERRY. Right, exactly. So across this country we don't value women. We don't have paid leave. We have to go back to work really quick, but we don't have child care so all those things impact our ability to have a healthy pregnancy. So how we then get into the hospital and need to rush out or if someone is doing something quickly, it makes it more difficult for us to live. So that happens really acutely for women of color and so you see that impact of implicit bias.

So what you can legislate is rules around training on implicit bias. What you can legislate is accountability for the entire system to look at every death and make sure that all the structures that they need to have in place are put there so there is not just one individual nurse or doctor but it is the entire structure.

Ms. DEGETTE. Yes, yes.

And Ms. Stewart, many nations have actually been able to cut the rate of maternal mortality in half. I talked about that in my opening statement. I wonder if you can give us some ways that they have been able to do that, that we can model our own behavior on in the U.S.

Ms. STEWART. Well, in many of those countries, Congresswoman, all of the outcomes relative to moms and babies are far better than they are here in the U.S. So one of the things about what is going on here in the United States is we are focusing on maternal mortality today as we should and maternal morbidity as we should. But if you look at all the outcomes around moms and babies, whether it is around premature birth, infant mortality, our outcomes are far worse than many other, most other developed countries in the world.

Ms. DEGETTE. And many underdeveloped countries too.

Ms. STEWART. And some in many underdeveloped, emerging countries. I mentioned in my opening statement our maternal mortality rates are worse than even countries like Slovenia and——

Ms. DEGETTE. So what are some of the things these countries have done?

Ms. STEWART. So I think it starts at the highest level of a policy environment and an environment that respects and cares for and prioritizes women and women's health and women and babies. So when you look at certain countries, Scandinavian countries for example, there are a range of policies that are far more supportive of women having a healthier lifestyle before being pregnant, having healthier pregnancies, and then having the kind of support even after pregnancy to make sure that they recover from their pregnancies well, that they feel supported, that they don't feel overwhelmed.

And we know the issues of stress in this country. Chronic stress, for example, can have a devastating impact on the health of women and the health of moms that impact not only them but their babies as well. So I think it starts with making sure that women have the healthcare coverage that they need, have access to the care we need. We have talked about that. Half of the pregnancies in this country are covered by Medicaid. We need to make sure that all women have the kind of coverage they need. We need to make sure there are services in their communities that are accessible as we mentioned earlier around the deserts that exist.

And then I think we need to make sure that postpartum, Medicaid doesn't stop within 60 days of delivering the baby. That it extends so that moms have the kind of care and health care and support that they need even as they recover from their pregnancies.

Ms. DEGETTE. Thank you. Thank you so much. I yield back, Mr. Chairman. Thanks to all of you.

Mr. BURGESS. The chair thanks the gentlelady. The chair recognizes the gentleman from Virginia, Mr. Griffith, 5 minutes for your questions, please.

Mr. GRIFFITH. Thank you very much, Mr. Chairman, and I thank our panelists for being here.

Mr. Johnson, I am just so sorry. Nobody should have to go through that. And of course I am sitting there while you are testifying thinking about my wife, her C-section with my first son. So I am very, very sorry. And as Ms. DeGette said, if there is anything that we can do I am sure we would try including passing this bill.

So here is a question for you all. I like the bill, and I like the bill because it will have us looking at it from a national perspective. If we just do it on a state perspective it may not work. Because I represent the corner of Virginia that is outside Appalachia and the Allegheny Highlands and so, I border four states.

The Bristol Herald-Courier did a series of articles last year on neonatal abstinence syndrome because we have a high number at the hospital in Tennessee, but those are my constituents even though they are going to a hospital in Tennessee. I believe that hospital serves at least three states. And so if you are looking at it from a state perspective, Virginia is going to look a whole lot better on substance abuse and other things than Ohio. But if you compare Ohio just with my section of the state, we are probably in pretty good similarity. We are in sync along with West Virginia because we have similar problems and similar backgrounds. And I have got to have some of the deserts on your map because I have an area that two of my counties have lost their hospitals.

And so, I want to see this data from a regional perspective not just a state perspective because my part of Virginia is not like Arlington or even Virginia Beach or Richmond. It is completely different and if you are just looking at it from a state perspective you get a skewed picture from my region. So I like the bill.

So then the questions become, do we overload the bill, and you don't want to do that. Sometimes you can put too much on it. Do we overload it by trying to include prenatal and neonatal care into the study? If we don't and if Ms. Beutler is in agreement, I would say expand it. If it is going to overload it and we might not get it passed by the end of the year, let's get this one passed and do something else.

But how, Ms. Stewart, how do we fix it? I am a big advocate of telemedicine. Obviously can't deliver the baby by telemedicine, but maybe some prenatal or pre-birth care, some neonatal care could be done that way. What do you think of that?

Ms. STEWART. Yes. Actually, we think the prospects of telemedicine especially for prenatal care can be very exciting and very productive. There have been several studies to show that women in rural areas, in urban areas, low-income women are very comfortable actually receiving care. And we also know that in the postpartum, we have some programs going on right now in the postpartum stages where uploading data, checking, taking blood pressure at home, uploading that data has actually reduced maternal deaths significantly in places like Philadelphia and can do the same in rural areas.

So we think the aspect of telemedicine in this space can be extremely helpful to overcome some of the gaps and barriers that we have. I will say that we, for sure, believe very strongly that this area and the period of time postpartum is the most critical period for this bill and for these issues that we are talking about. So whatever we can do to make sure that women have the care they need during that period.

We are measuring maternal deaths up to a year, so we need to make sure that women have the support they need after the baby. We are rightfully so, and we still need to focus prenatal, but what we are talking about now is the care postpartum that is now so critical and is contributing to so many of these deaths. So thank you for raising these issues.

Mr. GRIFFITH. Thank you all for being here. I think as technology moves forward we may have different answers, but I do think we have to embrace everything we can for those areas that are under-served or have deserts as you call it. And I appreciate you all being here. Thank you all so much for what you do and I yield back.

Mr. BURGESS. The chair thanks the gentleman. The gentleman yields back. The chair recognizes the gentlelady from Florida, Ms. Castor, 5 minutes for questions, please.

Ms. CASTOR. Well, thank you, Mr. Chairman, for holding this very important hearing on maternal mortality. And I really want to thank my colleague, Diana DeGette, and Congresswoman Herrera Beutler, for their work on the Preventing Maternal Deaths Act. And thank you to all of the witnesses who, you all have all devoted your careers to this, and Mr. Johnson, I take your story to heart especially.

This is a long overdue hearing and I do hope that this is just a start on an important focus on policy regarding maternal health because I don't believe that most people in the United States of America today understand that we are not doing so well. That women in the United States are more likely to die from childbirth or pregnancy-related causes than women in other parts of the developed world. That is not acceptable and the racial disparities are particularly disturbing. In Florida, we have our Pregnancy-Associated Mortality Review committee. In Tampa we are home to at the University of South Florida, the Lawton and Rhea Chiles Center for Healthy Mothers and Babies, and I have some wonderful experts there who help me. They have shared with me the latest Florida pregnancy-related mortality rates.

Since 1999, Florida's pregnancy-related mortality rate has been flat with no significant trend. How can that be that since 1999 things have not gotten better? I just, I think that is outrageous.

The committee found that hemorrhage-related deaths are the leading cause of pregnancy-related deaths in Florida by far. And of course we know that more than half of these deaths are preventable. Florida's most recent review committee has the statistics for 2016. They have identified 157 pregnancy-associated deaths, 21 died during the postpartum period. That has been the focus of many of your remarks.

Dr. Coslett-Charlton, I understand in May that ACOG released a number of recommendations on ways to optimize postpartum care for mothers including that new moms should have contact with their OB/GYN or other obstetric care provider within 3 weeks postpartum in a comprehensive, postpartum visit no later than 12 weeks after birth. Why is focusing on that fourth trimester or postpartum period important for the health of new moms and what are the barriers? We talked a little bit about it, but let's go into greater detail. What are the barriers that you and your colleagues see to prioritizing the fourth trimester? Transportation, child care—give us a little update on that.

Dr. COSLETT-CHARLTON. So that is a wonderful question and that is one of the exciting things that ACOG has developed, like you said, over the past several months is reevaluating the fourth trimester or postpartum care. And we know that when we look at preventable deaths that about half of those preventable deaths occur within that year within delivery.

So it is really important that we continue to engage patients on the importance of postpartum care and also reduce those barriers that you are discussing. Number one being access, number two being, in Pennsylvania I am fortunate to practice in a state that I did residency and medical school and practice in Pennsylvania, and in Pennsylvania when you are pregnant you are covered. And I cannot imagine a woman not being covered during pregnancy. But that coverage for Medicaid patients ends at 6 weeks postpartum and we know that things can happen afterwards.

And it isn't just the issues with—I have had plenty of women have preeclampsia or hypertensive disorders that need very close follow up. I have seen women seize 6 weeks after delivery in the emergency room related to preeclampsia. So those identification of patients that are at risk, number one. Number two, having important communications in a manner such as telemedicine within the first several weeks after delivery and especially in high-risk patients is critical.

And also, we talk a lot about postpartum depression and mental health disorders and how important it is that we screen women adequately and continue screening and keeping them within that period and also educating patients of the importance of the postpartum period. And we think that that might come during the prenatal period and that we need to do work to emphasize the importance of postpartum to women when they are having their babies because, I am a mother of four children.

I am embarrassed to say it. I don't know if I went back for a postpartum visit. I know I am an obstetrician and I know that, are privy to knowing the signs, but I was caring for children and having important maternal and parental leave, it is very important having the transportation. So there are so many policy things that are exciting and that, going forward hopefully we can look to all of you to make those favorable changes a reality.

Ms. CASTOR. Yes. One of the major gaps I see in my state and other states, Florida is in the minority of states that did not expand Medicaid. And I worry about the continuity of care for young families, for young women especially if they are not taking care of themselves early on and then they reach a gap after they have their baby. Has Medicaid been expanded long enough for there to be any studies on the differences on maternal mortality in states that have expanded Medicaid and states that have not, do you all know?

Dr. PERRY. I know for health in general, but not specifically maternal mortality and that is why this bill will be really helpful for us to be able to drill down on more details on maternal mortality.

Ms. CASTOR. Thank you very much and I yield back.

Mr. GRIFFITH [presiding]. The gentlelady yields back. The gentleman from Missouri, Mr. Long, is recognized for 5 minutes.

Mr. LONG. Thank you, Mr. Chairman. And I have heard a lot of testimony over my years on the committee here and, Mr. Johnson, I don't know that I have ever heard any more heartfelt or any more important testimony that what we heard from you here today. So thank you for being here and I know it is hard to do, and but hopefully your voice will add a voice and will garner more attention to this, so thank you for being here.

A quick question for you, your first son, was that—I understand that was a C-section also?

Mr. JOHNSON. Yes, sir. That was a C-section.

Mr. LONG. Was that a planned C-section like the next one or an emergency?

Mr. JOHNSON. No, that was not. So that was an emergency C-section so we went in for, we didn't expect it and so that was part of the reason that the C-section was recommended during the delivery of Langston, our second son.

Mr. LONG. OK, OK. Because I am curious, but yes, I am a little familiar with the emergency part of that situation, so yes.

Ms. Stewart, I just want to thank you for what you do at March of Dimes and the big event you hold every year here in Washington, D.C. The cook-off I call it. What is the official name of it?

Ms. STEWART. It is called a Gourmet Gala.

Mr. LONG. That is what I was going to say if you hadn't interrupted me.

Ms. STEWART. It is a lot of good food there.

Mr. LONG. Gourmet Gala.

Ms. STEWART. Gourmet Gala.

Mr. LONG. It is a dandy and it raises a lot of money every year for March of Dimes and I appreciate that.

Ms. STEWART. Absolutely. And we appreciate all of your support for that. Thank you.

Mr. LONG. Right. Dr. Coslett-Charlton, as you note, only 33 states have a maternal mortality review committee, many of which are newly created. Could you talk about the important role the Centers for Disease Control and Prevention is giving technical assistance to states to either help them establish MMRCs or ensure that they are operating effectively and getting appropriate data?

Dr. COSLETT-CHARLTON. I would be happy to speak of that. As the state that has a very newly formed committee, I mentioned earlier that our MMRC is meeting for the first time at the end of October and I am very excited to see the outcomes of our getting together and being able to collect this data effectively. The CDC Foundation has actually reached out to us and has been integral in not only determining the makeup of the committee and working well with our Department of Health and members of the committee, but also ensuring again standardization and by knowing best practices from other states. So having that cooperation is essential.

The other thing is that through the CDC there are data collecting tools, the MMRIA, collecting tools which will standardize the reporting part of the MMRCs so that we would be able, if the reports are looking different from every state it is a difficult task to try to come to a consensus. So we keep talking about the importance of making sure we keep standardization and the support through the CDC with the MMRIA application is an excellent example of that.

Mr. LONG. OK. In your testimony you discuss Pennsylvania's efforts to establish MMRC this year. What has been your experience so far in getting it up and running?

Dr. COSLETT-CHARLTON. Well, fortunately we have an extremely supportive Department of Health for this issue and some of it has been similar to our efforts here is recognizing that there is a problem. And some of the national attention to the problem has really given some interest to members that have been very interested in participating in this bill.

Our bill was supported unanimously—House, Senate, and by the Governor's Office. So this was an easy ask at this time, but it really, it was more momentum initiative and a lot of the reports coming out that this truly is a problem that, you know, opened the eyes of many and we realized that we need to tackle this. And it is not a hard thing to tackle if you do it the right way and there are best practices already established.

Mr. LONG. And getting data on why pregnancy-related deaths are happening is essential of course, but what can we do to improve outcomes once we receive that data and can you talk about the role MMRCs have once that data is collected?

Dr. COSLETT-CHARLTON. So some of collecting the data is important so that we can use it to see where it needs not only nationally but also in communities. And we talk about these perinatal collaboratives that the CDC and the national effort to collect data will be the mothership and hopefully we will be able to send out the tentacles to go out in the communities and find where there is deficiencies and where there is disparities and do better to be able to connect patients and meet those needs and to hopefully a realization where access really is an issue.

Maternity care is difficult to deliver and, we talk even about Philadelphia that has closed half of its maternity hospitals in the past decade. The only hospitals that are delivering right now are university institutions because a lot of hospitals find the reimbursement not adequate for the care and liability exposure and a multitude of things which is not for the conversation here.

But it is really important that we are able to identify where these deserts are—I think that is wonderful—in care and be able to improve upon that.

Mr. LONG. OK, thank you. And once again thank you all very much for being here. I appreciate your time in taking time out of your day and week to come up here and testify. And, Mr. Chairman, I yield back.

Mr. BURGESS. The gentleman yields back. The chair thanks the gentleman. The chair recognizes the gentlelady from Illinois, Ms. Schakowsky, 5 minutes for questions, please.

Ms. SCHAKOWSKY. Thank you. I want to join my colleagues who have thanked you so much for this, all of you. I want to thank you, Mr. Johnson, for turning this tragedy into something positive. It took a lot of courage and probably a lot of time away from being a dad. And so I just want to express my appreciation to all of you and just mention that in particular.

I think that the WHO and the CDC reports, et cetera, were really a wake-up call for people. I have been aware of communities near me, in Milwaukee for example, where we have seen this rise in maternal mortality, infant mortality as well, and it has really been unacceptable that we in a country, the richest country in the world, would see these kinds of results. It is really, it is absolutely shameful.

So I wanted to—and I think there are a lot of ways that we are failing mothers and children, especially African American women who are three to four times more likely to die from childbirth. We just simply have to do better. But I am concerned about the new proposals, the Trump Public Charge Rule that puts maternal and infant health in grave danger. By targeting legal taxpaying immigrants in this country, this rule seeks to discourage immigrants from using the government services that pay for—that are paid for with their tax dollars—Medicaid, CHIP, SNAP, WIC, and the Earned Income Tax Credit, just to name a few.

So let me ask Dr. Coslett-Charlton and Dr. Crear Perry, women who qualify for Medicaid that would cover pregnancy care and labor and delivery may face the impossible choice of jeopardizing their legal immigration status in this country or go without needed care. And let me just add that right now in my very diverse district, we are finding that people who qualify are not signing up for benefits, right now, because they are so fearful. So if women are forced to go without needed prenatal care, what could that mean to her health and risk of maternal mortality?

Dr. PERRY. So it is an opportunity for us to use the same empathy we have when we talked earlier about with the opioid addiction moment we are having where we don't want to criminalize moms who are addicted to opioids so we ensure that they have access to health care. If we criminalize women for using SNAP or Medicaid, we are also harming their ability to have a healthy pregnancy.

So we should be able to use that same feeling of empathy for all mothers that everyone who is in the United States deserves to have a healthy pregnancy and a healthy baby and so how do we make sure that they don't miss their prenatal care? For example, in Louisiana we didn't for a long time cover immigrant mothers and after Katrina it was a big push of new immigrants.

Ms. SCHAKOWSKY. This is even legal.

Dr. PERRY. Yes. And so we had to add that to the bill when we got more citizens coming because it was important for us to ensure that the babies had access and the babies had care. We saw an uptick in baby——

Ms. SCHAKOWSKY. But this would prohibit even citizen children of those parents from getting the benefits.

Dr. PERRY. Right. So we have to think about what are value is, right, so if we don't value citizen children, what do we value? If we don't think it is important for them to have treatment from a physician then what are we asking for as a country. So it is just we have to think about our own values as a country.

Ms. SCHAKOWSKY. I agree.

Yes, Doctor.

Dr. COSLETT-CHARLTON. And I would just like to add, ACOG strongly opposes any efforts to provide any barriers to any kind of care for pregnant women and postpartum and prenatal, and this rule obviously would do such. So and as a practitioner too, the woman is going to deliver the baby no matter what, so she is going to deliver. No matter what she is going to deliver. And, it is common sense that she needs prenatal care or, for fear of having rising morbidities and mortalities related to this.

Ms. SCHAKOWSKY. Yes, go ahead.

Ms. STEWART. I was going to say, Congresswoman, we have made a strong statement against that Public Charge Rule as well.

Ms. SCHAKOWSKY. Thank you. And I yield back. Thank you so much, all of you.

Mr. BURGESS. The chair thanks the gentlelady. The gentlelady yields back. The chair recognizes the gentleman from Florida, Mr. Bilirakis, 5 minutes for your questions, please.

Mr. BILIRAKIS. Thank you, Mr. Chairman. I appreciate it. Thanks for holding this very important hearing.

Ms. Stewart, as a parent I remember the birth of my children was such a joyful event. The idea that rates of maternal mortality are on the rise is horrifying as far as I am concerned. In our state it is on the rise. I read that women are dying from hemorrhage complications in the State of Florida. How does the Preventing Maternal Deaths Act help reverse the trend of women who are losing their lives to these typical medical complications?

Ms. STEWART. Well, I will defer to my medical colleagues to describe the issues around hemorrhage and how it is contributing, but I will say that what this bill is designed to do is to establish across the country maternal mortality review committees that are designed to collect data on every maternal death and to make sure that every state understands the underlying causes of death for each woman that dies as a result of childbirth.

But even beyond that what it is designed to do is to not just collect the data but to help states and to help the participants and the healthcare system design interventions that can actually eliminate deaths in the future.

And that is one of the things that is really important about this bill is not only collecting the data, but then designing interventions.

And of course if we collect data consistently across the country and if the sharing of interventions can also be shared we can certainly accelerate our ability to reduce and even eliminate maternal deaths. I will give you a couple of examples of how collecting data in MMRCs has been really helpful.

In Colorado, for example, data was collected and what was found is that women that experienced maternal death had also been experiencing suicide and depression and they were, in Colorado, able to find and identify where there were gaps in mental health services and actually close those gaps and give more mental healthcare services to women where they needed it.

In Ohio, they actually did something, which I think is really important, which is do additional training for hospital staff beyond just the doctors themselves, hospital staff where they went through simulations of training in obstetrical emergency situations so that they could actually be more responsive in the event of an emergency situation.

So MMRCs are not only about collecting the data, but actually putting into action the things that can actually eliminate maternal deaths. And that is why this bill is so important and that is why a national bill and a national effort is also so important, so the data can be consistent, can be collected, we can see the data, we can actually track the interventions more successfully.

Mr. BILIRAKIS. Thank you very much for that answer.

Dr. Coslett-Charlton, according to the Centers for Disease Control and Prevention, it lists indicators. Severe maternal morbidity has steadily been increasing in the years. What are the key drivers of this increase and how can it be addressed?

Dr. COSLETT-CHARLTON. Well, some things are recognizing and be able to maintain proper prenatal care and care of women throughout their reproductive years and identifying comorbidities such as, we talk about obesity and smoking cessation and where we see a rise in comorbidities with heart disease. So having active interventions before a pregnancy we find is critical to having a healthy labor and delivery for all women.

Mr. BILIRAKIS. So you feel that they are increasing. In this day and age with all the technology we have or is it just that we are getting more data on this or there definitely are increases in maternal deaths?

Dr. COSLETT-CHARLTON. Well, so far that is part of the purpose of this review is so that we were talking earlier about the accuracy of the data. So some speculation has been made that perhaps because for the past 5 years we were actually recording on death certificates whether or not a woman was pregnant when she died, or within a year after delivery whether or not that has caused a rise in the actual numbers that we are seeing. But when comparing to other countries that have had similar checkboxes on their certificates where they have seen a stabilization or a decrease, we have actually seen an increase.

So these committees are really imperative to really, exactly what you are saying, really know and be able to assess and accurately determine if those disease entities as well as maternal death if there is a change and make sure that we have accurate data so that we can successfully portray appropriate interventions.

Mr. BILIRAKIS. Yes, exactly. So, whether it is increasing or what have you, we have to focus on the issue. There is no question.

And, Dr. Johnson, you have my sympathies. I was in the VA Committee so I didn't get a chance to hear your testimony, but I know how difficult it must be for you.

Let's see, Dr. Crear Perry, please, our maternal mortality data has been described again as limited, unreliable, and even embarrassing by top researchers. Do you agree with these characterizations? And I know, let's expand upon this. Are there concerns with the research community regarding the integrity of the data being collected in states? What are those concerns and how might they be addressed federally?

Dr. PERRY. That is me. That is OK. Hi.

Mr. BILIRAKIS. Oh, you are over here. I am sorry.

Dr. PERRY. And so it is important, Dave Goodman and the folks at CDC are doing a great job of doing the data. They have been doing it for a very long time. They have dedicated their life to it. And they have looked at if the increase is due to error in data versus if it is an increase, that is true, and all the studies so far have come back saying no, there is an increase and it is from the data.

And so the robustness with which the CDC is working on to look at this issue is something that we should all value. And if they are part of this bill, they are not here testifying, but CDC is really integral to getting this work done and it is important that we understand that they are—that yes, there have been researchers that have given us pushback around the data over the years, but we have gotten better and better and this is just another way to get even more clear about how women are dying, because beginning at a granular level and look at the hospital level what is happening.

So yes, there have been a lot of articles about the data, but we truly know through the CDC that the rates are increasing and that we can do something together to do it better with this bill.

Mr. BILIRAKIS. Very good. Thank you and I yield back, Mr. Chairman.

Mr. BURGESS. The chair thanks the gentleman and the gentleman yields back.

The chair would just make the observation that I believe it was Dr. Callaghan from the CDC who came and spoke at one of our roundtables about a year ago. And you are correct. They are very thorough and they have been at this for a long time. They have a lot of good insights.

The chair recognizes the gentleman from Massachusetts, Mr. Kennedy, 5 minutes for your questions, please.

Mr. KENNEDY. Thank you, Mr. Chairman. I want to also thank you for your obviously lifelong and personal dedication to this issue given your profession before coming to Congress and still the work that you do. I want to also thank Representative Herrera Beutler who was here earlier and obviously our distinguished panel for joining us.

Mr. Johnson, excuse me. I will apologize. I have been in and out. Your words are extremely powerful, sir. Kira sounds like quite a woman. I have two kids under 3. I was in a delivery room about 9 months ago. Thoughts are with you and your family, sir.

In 2018, the United States of America has the highest rate of maternal deaths in the developed world. Every single year we mourn roughly 700 mothers who are lost to complications during their pregnancy, and at least 350 of those deaths are preventable. Most alarmingly, profound racial disparities exist in these statistics. Black women today are three to four times more likely to die of pregnancy or delivery complications than white women.

Before we try to explain that away on socioeconomic terms, just access to care, access to education, and higher income, we have to be clear that even when you control for those factors a wealthy black woman with an advanced degree is still more likely to die or to have a baby die than a poor white woman without a high school diploma. In the United States, a black woman is 22 percent more likely to die from heart disease than a white woman, 71 percent more likely to die from cervical cancer. Those are haunting statistics, but they still pale in comparison to the one we discussed here today, for black women are 243 percent more likely to die from pregnancy or childbirth-related causes: 243 percent. So we can't have a discussion about how to address a larger crisis in maternal mortality without having a discussion about how to confront the pervasive, systemic inequities that are buried deep within our system of health care in America.

And the last point I have to make is this, that there are, as we speak, 20 Republican Attorneys General that are attempting to repeal the Affordable Care Act in our court system after most of my Republican colleagues have voted to do the very same thing more times than I can count. So let's remember 9.5 million. That is the number of previously uninsured women that gained healthcare coverage including maternity care which is an essential health benefit under the Affordable Care Act. Coverage for women of color grew at more than twice the rate of women overall in 2013 to 2015. So to have a conversation about maternal mortality at a time when my Republican colleagues are using every tool in the book to roll back access to guaranteed maternal care and maternal coverage is a bit much.

And with that I want to direct my questions to Dr. Crear Perry and by the work that you have done, Doctor, in discussing how we need to move away from seeing race as a risk factor in maternal health and call the real risk factor what it is: racism. So can you extrapolate that a bit for the committee and, specifically, what do you believe to be the leading cause of those racial disparities I mentioned in maternal mortality rates?

Dr. PERRY. So we have done quite a bit of focus groups and work in hospitals around how patients feel disrespected and not heard and not listened to and not valued. And, a great example of that is Serena Williams, right. She gives an amazing story around how she had symptoms. She knew who she was. She is a very wealthy and healthy person as well and she still was not heard or valued.

So what we miss in this country is really being honest about when you don't see someone as being fully equal to you, you are less likely to think about their care in a very serious manner. You are less likely to address their issues in a serious manner, and you are less likely to spend the time that they need ensuring that they are healthy.

And so what we have to be able to do is have some truth around that conversation first and not act as if that is not a true——

Mr. KENNEDY. And so is there data that you would point to on this or is this something that is a bit bigger than fits into an Excel spreadsheet and a pie chart and how——

Dr. PERRY. This is going to be both a policy fix and a cultural shift, right. Like we have had policy shifts. We have had the civil rights movement, we have a lot of things of policy we can have, but as long as the culture still believes that black people are less valuable or inferior, and women, we are going to keep having the same conversations over and over and over again. So we have to have both a policy conversation and a culture shift.

Mr. KENNEDY. Anybody else want to comment on that? Mr. Johnson?

Mr. JOHNSON. So just talking about this from a personal experience and having an African American, extremely vibrant woman who was not in good health but in exceptional health at one of the top hospitals in the world, and to be quite honest with you, when this first happened and I was asked a question, do you think that this would have been different if your—do you think this is because your wife was black, or do you think the outcome would have been different if your wife was Caucasian, I was in so much pain I couldn't process that and the thought that the color of my wife's skin contributed to her death?

But what I am clear about is that she was not seen or valued as human. She wasn't. And the people who were responsible for her care that I trusted with her care failed to look at her in the same way that they would their daughter or their sister or their mother. And the reality of the situation is I am asked the question and people sometimes, and, the more I have spent with wonderful groups like Black Mamas Matter and the more I look at the data, people— and I am very clear about this issue of implicit bias and the contributing factors or racism. And people say you are making it a racial issue. I didn't make it a racial issue, the statistics did.

So what we have got to do is figure out how these women are valued and looked at as human, because what I said at night, thinking about my wife and I have to think about that question about would she be here today if she was Caucasian? Let me be clear that this is an epidemic that affects all families from all backgrounds and all walks of life, and unfortunately I know that personally because I have talked to these families and I have become very close to some of these fathers and some of these families and they are from all walks of life.

But we cannot address this issue without head-on facing the way that it is disproportionately and horrifyingly affecting African American mothers.

Mr. KENNEDY. Thank you, sir.

Chairman, thank you for the extra time. Thank you all for being here.

Mr. BURGESS. The chair thanks the gentleman. The gentleman yields back. The chair recognizes the gentleman from Georgia, Mr. Carter, 5 minutes for your questions, please.

Mr. CARTER. Thank you very much, Mr. Chairman, and thank all of you for being here. And, Mr. Johnson, thank you for your efforts and your work on this especially, and I echo the comments of all of my colleagues here today. We appreciate your courage.

Mr. Chairman, I believe this hearing was set for another time and I requested and I am sure others did that it be delayed so that we could have it. It is important to me and I am sorry if it disrupted any of you all or inconvenienced you.

But I am from the State of Georgia. In 2010, there was an Amnesty International report that flagged Georgia as being the number one state in maternal mortality. And that is why I expressed to the chairman, Mr. Chairman, I want to be at this hearing because this is real to me. In fact, when I served in the Georgia State Legislature and we passed Senate Bill 273 that created the MMRC and put it into the Georgia Department of Public Health.

And I wanted to ask you, Dr. Perry, because when we created that, you know, we followed the guidelines and we did what we were supposed to do. But I believe that your group was involved in a study, When the State Fails: Maternal Mortality and Racial Disparity in Georgia; so you are familiar with that?

Dr. PERRY. Yes, sir.

Mr. CARTER. I know you are. And I had the chance to look at it and study it and one of the things that it pointed out was the racial disparity in Georgia was the fact that even though the four categories—access to and quality of care, insurance access and pricing funding, and accountability around data analysis and use, even though we had those in there we are still failing on those, particularly access.

And my question is, what can we do? Tell me what I can take back to my state because this is important to me. I served in legislature. I was in Health and Human Services, vice chair of that committee, and I helped with this legislation. If, and the point has been made by my colleagues today, what can we do legislatively, but what can I do? What can I take back to the State of Georgia?

Dr. PERRY. Thank you so much. And I do work with Dr. Lindsay and the folks at Grady around the Georgia work and they are specifically trying to look at their mental healthcare service structure. So supporting mental healthcare services in Georgia is important. Supporting Medicaid expansion in Georgia is important. Supporting rural hospital closures in

Georgia is in support and like supporting support systems that include midwives and doulas in Georgia is important.

All the social structures that we see, all the states where we allow for us to disinvest in women honestly have poor outcomes. Even though you can look and do the study and see, we are working on things inside of hospitals because you have some great doctors in Georgia. You have some phenomenal people and some nurses and midwives. But until we build a structure that holds the entire state together, right, like from rural Georgia from—then we are not going to be able to see an improvement and we are being separated around ideals that don't allow us to come together. And it is important that we know we value all the moms in Georgia, rural moms, urban, they all need access to insurance.

Mr. CARTER. Well, thank you for mentioning that because as you well know, knowing the state we have a disparity between rural and urban.

Dr. PERRY. Exactly.

Mr. CARTER. I mean to say Georgia is Atlanta and everywhere else. So it really is.

Dr. PERRY. Exactly.

Mr. CARTER. Well, another part of that study that I was very interested in, because I am a big advocate of this, is the proposition that the state could develop ways to help religious organizations in leadership engage and advocate for quality health education and services.

And I am really big with wanting to include the religious community. And can you give me examples of how we can do that or examples of how that has worked before?

Dr. PERRY. Including, because if you think about mental health it is a great example, right, so a lot of religious organizations have access to therapy, access to group places where women can come to make sure they have grievance counseling.

So there has been a lot of work that religious organizations are there to be a safety net and a support for women. They can't replace medical care, but they can serve as a safety net. They can provide transportation. They can help with child care. Like all these other things that we are looking for that a community provides, because we know that women who have access to a community and to each other, the connectedness, have better outcomes.

So how do we create connectedness and community across this country and across Georgia.

Mr. CARTER. Right. And one last question and this could go to just about any of you. But the thing that I am wondering here is I know we are accumulating the data and we are, and I believe you said earlier the data is going to CDC. Are they crunching the science of it? Can we tie anything into this genetically, regionally?

Ms. STEWART. I will try and then others. CDC has had a surveillance system in place for a number of decades and thankfully we are able to collect a lot of data mainly coming from death certificates. And just recently now, death certificates now include whether or not a woman was pregnant within the last year, and so that information has been helpful.

But what we don't get from all of that—and by the way that voluntary system, CDC asks states around the country to voluntarily submit the data. There are epidemiologists that then review the data and we learn as much as we can from death certificates. But what we don't understand is that a death certificate does not necessarily tell the full story of how a woman may have died and what were the underlying causes and what were the potential interventions that could have been in place to prevent that.

And that is what this is about is taking the data we collect, improving it, improving the collection, making it consistent, having committees that then can design interventions and having them well-funded so that they can actually see meaningful improvement over time. So that is the difference.

Mr. CARTER. Good. Again, thank all of you. And, Mr. Johnson, thank you and God bless you.

Mr. JOHNSON. And I would just like to say that I am actually a native of Georgia and currently——

Mr. CARTER. Did this happen in Georgia?

Mr. JOHNSON. It actually happened in California but I am a native of Georgia.

Mr. CARTER. OK.

Mr. JOHNSON. Kira grew up in Decatur, Georgia and I grew up in East Point and we are back living in Georgia.

Mr. CARTER. Right.

Mr. JOHNSON. So we look forward to working together with you—

Mr. CARTER. Absolutely.

Mr. JOHNSON [continuing]. To see how we can help out too.

Mr. CARTER. Can I ask you, was your wife originally from Georgia?

Mr. JOHNSON. Absolutely. Decatur, Georgia. Born and raised.

Mr. CARTER. OK, see this is the point I am getting at here. We are the Cardiac Belt. Has anybody looked at any of this to kind of try to tie this into it?

Ms. STEWART. There is a lot of work being done on what is going on that is that are sort of the underlying causes to why so many women of color especially are dying, and there are a bunch of issues. I will mention one of them. By the way I am from Atlanta too. Don't hold that against me.

Mr. CARTER. I see a pattern here.

Ms. STEWART. We have known each other a long time.

Look, there is a very important study and we could go through a laundry list of things, but there is a very important study that has really helped all of us understand what are some of the underlying causes to why we see so many disparities among African American women in particular.

A study that was done by a researcher who is now at the University of Michigan but she started this study in New Jersey, I believe, where she started to look at this as your weathering. The fact that African American women's health tends to, and African American women tend to have more challenges the older they get, challenges in pregnancy, challenges in childbirth, challenges maybe post childbirth may be due to this issue of weathering, which is that the impact of chronic stress that may be coming from racism and discrimination over a long period of time.

This issue of weathering which tends to deteriorate one's health may be a big contributor why we see so many disparities. The fact that women are getting, are older as they are getting pregnant and the fact that if black women are older having babies and they are experiencing this impact from this weathering effect that that could explain in part why we are seeing so many outcomes.

Having said that, we still need to address the fact that we don't specifically have to accept that that is the case, we can actually do something about it. We can actually address those issues. We can actually deal with the underlying stress that exists. We can actually deal with the systems that may be creating the stress in the first place, and we can make sure that we understand when interventions are really effective across all communities.

Mr. CARTER. Thank you, Mr. Chairman. I yield back.

Mr. BURGESS. As the gentleman's time has expired, the chair recognizes the long-suffering Mr. Engel from New York, 5 minutes for your questions, please.

Mr. ENGEL. Thank you, Mr. Chairman. I appreciate those words, thank you.

Thank you, Mr. Chairman, for holding today's hearing. Just in listening, it is just shocking that right here in the United States women are dying from preventable pregnancy-related complications. That alone is shocking, but that women are more likely to die from those complications here than in other parts of the developed world, that is shocking. And the fact that this risk is three to four times higher for black women than white women, that is shocking.

So it is a tragedy and it is an emergency, and thank you, Mr. Johnson, for sharing your story with us.

I want to thank my colleagues, Congresswoman Herrera Beutler and Congresswoman DeGette, for introducing the Preventing Maternal Death Act legislation which I am a proud cosponsor of. And I hope that after today our committee can move forward on solutions to this problem that we really need to move more quickly. It is long past time we acted to reverse this horrible trend once and for all.

So let me ask this question. I have long supported investments in family planning and reproductive health and I am particularly interested in the impact that such investments can have on maternal mortality. As the ranking member of a House Foreign Affairs Committee, I have seen that impact on a global scale. In fiscal year 2016 alone, U.S. investments in family planning worldwide provided contraceptive services and supplies to 27 million women and couples, which in turn helped to prevent 11,000 maternal deaths.

So let me ask Drs. Crear Perry and Coslett-Charlton, would you each explain why meeting unmet need for contraception helps to prevent maternal deaths?

Dr. PERRY. So there has been some data that shows that the safety and security you get from having access to family planning and not having to worry about if you are going to get pregnant again because you are not planning to be pregnant at that moment really decreases your stress and your weathering and ensures that you have a healthier pregnancy.

We know that we have looked at the states that have more supportive policies around family planning also have better infant mortality rates and better maternal mortality rates. So it is not a coincidence that when you invest in family planning and when you invest in infrastructure for moms and babies, you actually create a safety net where people can live longer and be healthier. So it is important that these policies that are created in this House improve the ability for moms and babies to live.

Dr. COSLETT-CHARLTON. And I would certainly echo that response. But also it has been shown that women that are able to plan their pregnancies by spacing intervals between pregnancies and having access to adequate contraception that it improves the safety. There is very clear data to show that it improves outcomes in pregnancy and delivery also.

Mr. ENGEL. So thank you. But along those lines, let me ask you if either of one of you would explain why women in the United States specifically have unmet need for contraception. By that I mean they want to use modern contraception but are not currently.

Dr. PERRY. Well, it is a state and local issue, usually, around access to family planning and reproduction and because when we allow that to be made state-based wide people's personal, you get gaps in what states pay for, things like sex education, what states allow for, things like having birth control inside of high schools.

Once again I will say for my great State of Louisiana, we struggle with getting sex education in the schools. We struggle with getting access to family planning for the people who actually need it very desperately. So I think in an attempt to make for a safe environment for our state sometimes we mislabel what safety looks like. Safety looks like having access to choice when it comes to your reproduction. And when you have that access to choice and information, you can have a safer pregnancy and a safer outcome.

Mr. ENGEL. Well, thank you. Obviously there is a lot more work to do on this front. Let me mention this. A December report from the Guttmacher Institute estimated that globally, "fully meeting the unmet need for modern contraception would result in an estimated 76,000 fewer maternal deaths each year." That is 76,000.

So I want to ask either one of you doctors to please, if you agree is it fair to say that improving access to contraception for American women could help address the rates of maternal death in the United States?

Dr. PERRY. Yes.

Dr. COSLETT-CHARLTON. Yes.

Mr. ENGEL. That is a loaded question, but I wanted to put it out on the record. I want to also take this opportunity to briefly talk about legislation. I have introduced with Congressman Stivers, the Quality Care for Moms and Babies Act. The legislation would bring together diverse stakeholders to identify care quality benchmarks for women and children in Medicaid and CHIP as well as fund new and existing maternity and infant care quality collaboratives.

These collaboratives bring together local stakeholders such as doctors and nurse midwives to best share the best practices in improved care for patients, and I am grateful to both the ACOG and March of Dimes for supporting this legislation.

And let me ask you, finally, both—let me ask perhaps Ms. Stewart. I will ask you this. Wouldn't you agree that we should be measuring and evaluating performances of Medicaid and CHIP caring for America's moms and babies as well as investing in perinatal quality collaboratives which work to implement maternal mortality review committee recommendations at the state level?

Ms. STEWART. Congressman, we are very involved across the country in perinatal collaboratives and they are very effective and we would very much support them. And I would just add at this point which is that 60 percent of all births are covered by Medicaid and that is a lot of women and a lot of babies.

And whatever we can do to make sure that the quality of care exists for those women as it does for women in the private insurance market to make sure we are collecting the kind of data to understand what is effective and what is not and that we are sharing that data across states, we would firmly support that.

Mr. ENGEL. Thank you. Thank you very much. Thanks, Mr.

Chairman.

Mr. BURGESS. And the gentleman's time has expired.

Seeing no additional members wishing to ask questions, I want to thank all of our witnesses again for being here today. I have some documents I need to read into the record, a statement for the record from Sean Blackwell, M.D.; momsrising.org; and Alexis Joy Foundation. I also have the September report for the Maternal Mortality and Morbidity Task Force from the state of Texas[21]; a letter from Dr. Gary Hankins who participated in one of our roundtables—Dr. Hankins is from the University of Texas Medical Branch in Galveston; and Dr. Cardenas had mentioned the Obstetric Hemorrhage Toolkit in California[22] and I do have a copy of that I am going to submit for the record.

Also, documents from the March for Moms; Postpartum Support Virginia; Association of Maternal & Child Health Programs; Heart Safe Motherhood; Massachusetts Child Psychiatry Access Program; a letter signed by 1,000 Days and other patient groups; Americans United for Life;

---

[21] The information has been retained in committee files and can be found at: https://docs.house.gov/meetings/IF/IF14/20180927/108724/HHRG-115-IF14-20180927-SD022.pdf.

[22] The information has been retained in committee files and can be found at: https://docs.house.gov/meetings/IF/IF14/20180927/108724/HHRG-115-IF14-20180927-SD023.pdf.

Alexis Joy Foundation; Nurse-Family Partnership; Preeclampsia Foundation; Society for Maternal and Fetal Medicine; a letter from Timoria McQueen Saba; American College of Surgeons; KSM Consulting[23]; more California PPH; SAP America; and Forbes Insight Study.

[The information appears at the conclusion of the hearing.]

And just to end on a somewhat positive note, my grandfather was an OB/GYN, an academic OB/GYN at McGill University in Montreal and practiced obstetrics during the decade of the 1930s when the maternal mortality fell from all-time highs to all-time lows, certainly indicative that if we put our minds to it, it has happened before, it can happen again.

Pursuant to committee rules, I remind members they have 10 business days to submit additional questions for the record. I ask the witnesses to submit their responses within 10 business days upon receipt of the questions. Without objection, the subcommittee is adjourned.

[Whereupon, at 12:23 p.m., the subcommittee was adjourned.] [Material submitted for inclusion in the record follows:]

MomsRising.org

Where moms and people who love them go to change our world

MomsRising HR 1318 Preventing Maternal Death Acts Hearing Testimony

Hello, my name is Smita Nadia Hussain. I am the Maternal Justice Campaign Director at Moms Rising, a national organization of over a million members, with members in every state in the country, who organize and advocate around issues that impact mothers, children, and families. As Director of our Maternal Justice campaign, I work on grassroots organizing and advancing policy efforts to address the maternal mortality/morbidity issues in our country, concentrating on the disparities

---

[23] The information has been retained in committee files and can be found at: https://docs.house.gov/meetings/IF/IF14/20180927/108724/HHRG-115-IF14-20180927-SD004.pdf.

Black women experience. In fact, Black women, no matter their education or income level, are 3-4 time more likely to experience maternal mortality and morbidity, one of the widest disparities in ali of women's health.

I urge you to move HR 1318 The Preventing Maternal Deaths Act forward in today's Subcommittee on Health hearing to enable this important piece of legislation to go to a vote by the House of Representatives.

Why is this legislation important? The ability to protect the health of mothers and babies in childbirth is a basic measure of a society's development. Yet, currently, the United States holds the worst record for maternal and infant mortality in the developed world, and maternal mortality continues to rise. Every year in the U.S., 700 to 900 women die from pregnancy or childbirth related causes, and some 65,000 nearly die.

American women are more likely to die from pregnancy-related complications than women in 45 other countries including the United Kingdom and much poorer nations like Libya and Kazakhstan. Additionally the data reveal major racial disparities in maternal mortality rates: Black women are three to four times more likely to die from pregnancy complications than white women, independent of age, parity, or education in our nation.

This legislation would establish a program to help states review maternal deaths; establish and sustain a maternal mortality review committee; develop a plan for health care provider education to improve maternal care, and improve information collection on maternal deaths to provide public disclosure of information on maternal mortality. It will help enable health systems to address the factors leading to the disproportionate deaths of Black mothers and put recommendations in place to begin addressing racial disparities that have been present and unchanged for decades.

These are some of the critical solutions needed to address our nation's maternal mortality and morbidity crisis.

We can fix this; women don't have to die from childbirth. According to a recent analysis by the CDC Foundation, nearly 60 percent of maternal deaths in the U.S. are preventable. Sixty percent. If we are able to decrease that number by even a fraction, thousands of mothers' lives could be saved.

At Moms Rising, we have repeatedly heard the stories of women who've almost lost their lives and from those who've lost loved ones to childbirth related causes. Stories such as Carissa, from Olympia, WA.

> "After 40 hours of labor and 6 hours pushing, [my daughter] was in fetal distress and I had to have an emergency c-section. If we hadn't had access to a good doctor, and appropriate care, we both would have died. As it is, she is my miracle, and I am so thankful we are here! Good prenatal care and access to the childbirth center are not optional. We live in the wealthiest country in history, and there is no excuse for moms and babies to die needlessly."

We can and must do better to ensure that births are as safe and healthy as possible for all mothers. We must all work to ensure that the health of women and their children are made a priority. Thank you very much for your time.

September 17, 2018

Chairman Michael C. Burgess, MD
Ranking Member Gene Green
Subcommittee on Health
Committee on Energy and Commerce
Washington, DC

RE: "Better Data and Better Outcomes: Reducing Maternal Mortality in the U.S."

Dear Chairman and Ranking Member Green:

I write to you on behalf of the upcoming hearing scheduled for September 27, 2018 on Maternal Mortality. I lost my wife Alexis Joy in 2013 due to postpartum suicide, and I deeply believe that Congress needs to be aware of this ongoing crisis.

On August 30th, 2013 my wife Alexis and I had our first child, a beautiful healthy baby girl we named Adriana Joy.

August 30th, 2013 was supposed to be the happiest day of our lives. Rather, it was the most challenging, eye opening, brutal reality we had never been prepared for. Our daughter's delivery was a code blue delivery. This was the beginning of the end of our perfect life as I knew it. Alexis was diagnosed with PTSD from the delivery. Breastfeeding proved way more challenging than either of us would have thought. Baby Adriana cried, a lot. This did not help our situation.

Alexis was diagnosed with PTSD. She started worrying over everything. "Our perfect baby might be damaged," Alexis thought. Alexis was convinced Adriana had brain damage and we took the baby in for testing on her brain. She was fine. This was an answer my wife couldn't accept. Her fears seemed to grow daily. Each day she became more irrational, paranoid, and cried more. She would push food around on her plate but never took a bite.

She had been calling her ObGYN, psychiatrist, and pediatrician during this entire period of time. Each one said "Don't worry, it's just the baby blues. It will pass. You're fine. Just relax and enjoy this time."

I watched my wife lose nearly 50 pounds in 30 days. One doctor in an emergency psychiatric unit pulled me aside and said "Your wife's not crazy. She will be fine. She just needs her family and friends. But, just in case there's only two ways women as pretty as her commit suicide. They either asphyxiate themselves in the garage or overdose on pills.

Just get rid of the car keys at your house and any prescription pills she could take. Women like her would never commit suicide in a "sloppy" way. They would never want to be remembered not looking their best."

In our struggles to find help for my wife Alexis, we went to 7 different hospitals or crisis centers in her last 13 days.

On the morning of October 8th, 2013 I woke up to our Maltese puppy named Lucy, frantically barking to wake me up. Something seemed off. The air was stale, it was almost as if time had stopped. It's a feeling you have to experience to really know. In that moment I knew. I jumped out of bed. Ran downstairs screaming Alexis name. No response. I could hear my daughter crying. I ran down to the kitchen, no Alexis. The dining room, family room, office- no Alexis. Outside on the deck, not there either. Downstairs to the garage, not there. In the basement, not there either. By this point I'm literally crazed, panicking screaming at the top of my lungs. I run back upstairs to find my daughter strapped to her changing table and crying. Still no Alexis. I run back downstairs to look again. As I look to the back of the basement there was my beautiful, perfect, love of my life. Lifeless hanging by TV cable from my basement ceiling. I called 911 screaming for them to help me save her. I remember going through the chest compressions and mouth to mouth bargaining with God please, please bring her back. Suddenly, paramedics and cops were everywhere. They pulled me from her and started working on her. This was only probably 7 minutes. The craziest 7 minutes nobody should ever go through.

These 7 minutes that paled in comparison to the 5 1/2 weeks of hell my wife had to endure. 7 minutes that pale in comparison to the eternity I will spend missing my best friend. 7 minutes that pale in comparison to the lifetime my daughter will spend wondering who her mom was. 7 minutes that pale in comparison to the times I spend coming up with answers to my daughter's questions about why her mommy died. Will my daughter blame herself someday?

Will she do the same thing when she has a baby someday? Will she even want to have a baby someday? 7 minutes that pale in comparison to the anxiety I get when my reality sets in that I have to do this parenting thing all alone.

All of this for no good reason.

Since my wife lost her battle with postpartum suicide, Pittsburgh has decided to not wait for another tragedy and to do something about it. Moms in Pittsburgh can now see a psychiatrist in under 48 hours because of Allegheny Health Network and Highmark Blue Cross Blue Shield and the Alexis Joy Foundation. I'm confident in the near future it will be under 24 hours.

PPD is not a women's health issue, it is a family health issue. I firmly believe we owe it to our children to fix this preventable and treatable problem. I know I will do my part to make sure my daughter gets the care she deserves if needed, someday.

As Congress takes into consideration the escalating rise in maternal mortality and the need to figure out "Why are Mothers dying in this great country," I implore Congress to take a look at the mental health aspect of this issue. Perhaps if there was enough information on maternal mental health, its risks and evidenced based treatment options, my wife would be here with me and our daughter, today.

I thank you for your time.

Sincerely,

Steven D'Achille, Founder
The Alexis Joy Foundation
Gibsonia, PA
www.alexisjoyfoundation.org

Alexis Joy
Foundation

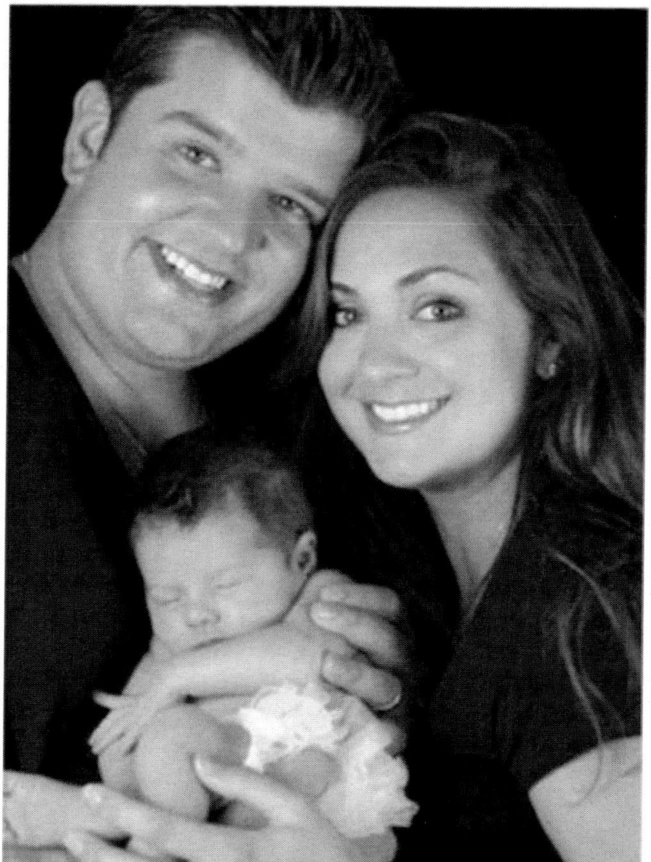

STATEMENT FOR THE RECORD, SEPTEMBER 27, 2018, HOUSE ENERGY & COMMERCE COMMITTEE, HEALTH SUBCOMMITTEE HEARING, BETTER DATA AND BETTER OUTCOMES: REDUCING MATERNAL MORTALITY IN THE U.S.

Submitted by:
Sean Blackwell, MD
President, Society for Maternal Fetal Medicine
Washington DC
Contact: Katie Schubert, Chief Advocacy Officer

Thank you for the opportunity to provide a statement for the record in support of bipartisan efforts to reduce a rising national maternal mortality rate in the United States. I submit this statement for the record on behalf of the Society for Maternal-Fetal Medicine, or SMFM.

SMFM was founded in 1977 as the medical professional society for high-risk obstetricians. Maternal-fetal medicine specialists treat high-risk pregnant women – women who have underlying medical conditions and become pregnant, women who develop life-threatening medical conditions as a result of becoming pregnant, or women whose fetuses do not develop normally and, in some cases, may become unviable. MFMs are obstetricians who have an additional three years of training and are on the front lines of these complicated pregnancy cases. Because we see these cases every day we are deeply concerned with our country's rising maternal morbidity and mortality rates.

Unfortunately, there is still much we do not know about why so many women are dying in childbirth or as a result of or following pregnancy. What we do know is that maternal mortality is just the tip of the iceberg and as many as half are potentially preventable. For each maternal death, there are numerous other women who suffer serious complications, what we refer to as severe maternal morbidities. We are working to understand more and do more to prevent these tragic outcomes.

What we do know is that we can do better. Despite advances in obstetrical care, the United States still trails the developed world in its maternal mortality rate. While the rate of maternal mortality has fallen in most developed nations, it is rising here. In a 2015 study, the United States had the highest maternal mortality rate at 26.4 deaths for every 100,000 live births, followed by the United Kingdom at 9.2 deaths for every 100,000 live births. That translates into 2 to 3 women dying each day in the United States at a time that should be one of the happiest in their lives and the lives of their families.

When obstetrical care is standardized – when all women receive certain interventions when faced with complications – outcomes improve. The state of California has demonstrated remarkable improvements in pregnancy outcomes by reviewing the death records of pregnancy and postpartum women and standardizing care and working systematically to implement standardized care based on what they learned. Specifically, the California Maternal Quality Care Collaborative, via the use of state-wide outreach collaboratives, has been able to reduce severe maternal morbidity by 20.8 percent between 2014 and 2016 among the hospitals that participate in maternal hemorrhage and preeclampsia best practices.[24] The United Kingdom has long had what is known as the Confidential Inquiry into Maternal Deaths. As a result of that program, standardized interventions were developed and implemented that have had a dramatic impact on reducing maternal deaths from conditions like venous thromboembolism.

We also know that with standardized data collection and review of maternal death cases, we can improve care and save lives. To assist with this, in September 2016, SMFM and the American College of Obstetricians and Gynecologists (ACOG) published an Obstetric Care Consensus outlining a process for identifying maternal cases that should be reviewed. We need better, more standardized data surrounding maternal mortality so that we can accurately attribute its causes and prevent it wherever possible. There are some new tools available to share knowledge – for example,

[24] https://www.cmqcc.org/qi-initiatives/obstetric-hemorrhage/hemorrhage-collaboratives.

with the support of the CDC Foundation, the Association of Maternal and Child Health Programs (AMCHP) created a web portal highlighting performing maternal mortality reviews so that states that have maternal mortality review committees can share information about best practices with states that are interested in setting up review committees. The National Network of Perinatal Quality Collaboratives sponsored by the Centers for Disease Control and Prevention and the March of Dimes was recently launched to provide support to state Perinatal Quality Collaboratives so that they can improve maternal and infant health outcomes. However, to accomplish this, they need more information about the problem that they are attacking.

Once we have data it will be important to translate that data into actionable recommendations that can be implemented on a state level. This last piece is critical if we truly want to move the needle on reducing maternal morbidity and mortality in the United States and ensuring healthy births, moms and babies. With technical assistance and support from the CDC, as provided for in HR 1318, the Preventing Maternal Deaths Act, states can expertly create and sustain maternal mortality review committees.

There is more that we can do together to reduce maternal mortality and severe maternal morbidity as healthcare providers. The establishment of maternal mortality review committees is just the first step. As an example, a focus on care coordination and the importance of considering social determinants of health in all of our solutions cannot be stated enough.

SMFM has endorsed HR 1318 and appreciates Representatives Herrera Beutler, DeGette and Costello's leadership on this important issue. With the bipartisan support and further leadership of Chairman Burgess, Ranking Member Green and the entire Health Subcommittee, as well as Chairman Walden, Ranking Member Pallone and the full Energy and Commerce Committee, we can take the first step in reducing maternal mortality.

No woman goes into pregnancy fearing a significant complication or death. Having a child should be a joyous time – but far too often complications arise and these impact not just the woman—but also her baby and her entire family. We can do more, and we must do more. With a state-based review process, better data, actionable recommendations and a focus on policies that are informed by findings from state-based review process and evidence, we can and will make a big difference. We urge you to support HR 1318 and move it forward to House floor action. Thank you again for providing me the opportunity to speak and for shining a light on this important issue.

School of Medicine, Department of Obstetrics & Gynecology
Gary D.V. Hankins, MD
Garland D Anderson, MD
Distinguished University
Chair in Obstetrics and Gynecology
Professor and Chairman

MEMORANDUM

Date: September 12, 2018
To: Congressman Michael Burgess
From: Gary D.V. Hankins, MD
Chairman, Department of OB/GYN

RE: Maternal Mortality Testimony

I greatly appreciate Congressman Michael Burgess providing me the opportunity to submit written testimony to the Health Subcommittee of the United States Congress. By way of introduction, I am currently the Chairman of Obstetrics and Gynecology at the University of Texas Medical Branch in Galveston, Texas where I have practiced for the last 22 years. Prior to coming to UTMB I was on active duty in the United States Air Force for 22 years, again serving a practicing obstetrician gynecologist. I am trained both as an OBGYN physician as well as having subspecialty training in Maternal Fetal Medicine and in Critical Care medicine.

Additionally, I most recently served as Vice Chair for the state of Texas Maternal Morbidity and Mortality Review Committee.

Having spent considerable time looking at maternal mortality in the United States, it is clear that substantial improvement is needed and should be accomplished. The mortality within the United States is more than twice that in other areas of the industrialized world and greater than 6 times that in Sweden. While it is unlikely that we could ever achieve the maternal mortality in the United States that can be achieved in a country as small as Sweden, it is clear to me that concentrating in the three areas that I will detail below, would substantially (I estimate by at least 50%) reduce maternal mortality in the United States.

1) Interpregnancy care; The provision of healthcare to many pregnant women within the United States, particularly those on government programs such as Medicaid, is episodic. That care begins only with the diagnosis of pregnancy and ends within a relatively short period following the conclusion of pregnancy. As such, women often enter into the pregnancy with uncontrolled or only partially controlled diabetes, hypertension, thyroid disease, and many other medical conditions. It is these complications of pregnancy which translate not only to a poor outcome for the women but also a poor outcome for the baby, often to include potential fetal malformations as well as premature deliveries. The cost burden of not providing pregnancy care and control of these chronic conditions is staggering and would greatly exceed the cost to control these diseases and conditions before the woman ever enters into pregnancy. As a specific example, failure to control Diabetes Mellitus carries a substantial risk that the fetus will have either a midline CNS developmental defect i.e., cleft lip, cleft palate, spina bifida, or a cardiac anomaly. These fetal malformations can be reduced to near zero if the diabetes is controlled prior to pregnancy. This is but one example of where dollars could be very well spent. The return on investment on quality of life and a reduction on long-term expenditures are very substantial.

2) Regionalization. The fact that regionalization of medical care to concentrate getting the patient to the appropriate level facility works has been demonstrated by the pediatricians and neonatologists for at least 30 years. It is largely through regionalization that the neonatal survival rates have been markedly increased at the same time that long term morbidity has been decreased for premature infants. This same model is applicable to pregnancy and the transfer of women with substantial complications to regional centers with the appropriate staffing! By way of one example, major maternal cardiac conditions should be sent to centers with specialized ability to provide care for these highly complex and complicated women. Such care is available through the input of teams of physicians with expertise to include maternal fetal medicine specialists, cardiologists, and intensivists to name a few. As an immediate first step towards reducing maternal mortality, the combination of providing interpregnancy care and regionalization of the care system hold the promise of significant immediate improvement in maternal mortality & morbidity.
3) Mental Health Services. In the review on the state of Texas Maternal Morbidity and Mortality Committee it was a surprise to me as a clinician that almost half of the deaths occurring were as a result of either a drug overdose or suicides/homicides. In the majority of these cases the women had either not been referred for mental health services or had not gained access to facilities capable of providing mental health services. It was clearly my misperception that the overwhelming majority of maternal deaths were as a result of the classic issues of obstetric hemorrhage, poorly controlled hypertension and/or infection as is still taught in many medical schools. To the contrary, almost half of maternal deaths relate to the mental health of the woman. Accordingly, while the first two strategies that I've outlined above *would* make a significant impact on the actual medical conditions, that would (at max) affect only about half of maternal deaths during pregnancy.

Attention to provision of mental healthcare when needed is essential.

I would conclude by briefly addressing the disparity in outcomes based upon race and ethnicity. There can be no debate but that the healthcare outcomes for the Native American population and for the African American population is far worse than for the Caucasian population. Similarly, the outcome for Hispanics, especially if first generation, actually exceeds that of Caucasians in the United States. Accordingly, specific populations are readily identified where a greater impact on the outcome certainly should be able to be achieved. I'd also point out that throughout the United States even in those states with the lowest maternal mortality, this disparity in outcomes persist and sometimes is even worse. Finally & sadly, the disparities in these outcomes based upon race and ethnicity is the absolute worst in our Nation's Capital.

I want to thank Dr. Burgess and the committee for allowing me to express my thoughts on this issue. I commend you for undertaking this difficult task and stand ready to assist you in any fashion I might.

Regards,

Gary DV Hankins, MD
September 11, 2018
TO: US House Energy & Commerce Committee

WRITTEN TESTIMONY OF THE MARCH FOR MOMS ASSOCIATION AT A HEARING OF THE HOUSE COMMITTEE ON ENERGY AND COMMERCE SUBCOMMITTEE ON HEALTH ON THE "MATERNAL MORTALITY ACT" (H.R. 1318)

Dear Committee Members, On behalf of the March for Moms Association Board of Directors, we value your time and our opportunity to highlight key issues related to maternal mortality in the United States. March for Moms Association, now in its second year, is a growing, multi-stakeholder coalition sharing like-minded urgency to improve the wellbeing of mothers in the US.

We established March for Moms in 2017 to address a widespread crisis among American families during the universally vulnerable period that stretches from pregnancy through delivery of a baby to early parenthood. Right now, Americans who are starting or growing their families face starkly greater risks than their parents did.

> In just one generation, the odds of an American mother dying from a pregnancy-related cause has increased by more than 50%, a risk that is consistently three to four times higher for black mothers than white mothers.
>
> For every death, there are 100 mothers who experience life-threatening injuries. For every injury, there are tens of thousands of mothers who experience avoidable suffering in the form of physical or mental illness, professional disruption, and/or wider societal disempowerment.

Our inclusion of two graphs depict the current state and worsening trend of maternal health childbirth in our country. The first graph published this month from AHRQ illustrates severe maternal morbidity from 2006-2015. Severe maternal morbidity is defined as including unexpected outcomes of labor and delivery that result in significant short- or long-term consequences to a woman's health. Often called near-misses, deliveries involving severe maternal morbidity generally include life-threatening conditions, such as acute myocardial infarction, pulmonary embolism, or sepsis. Severe maternal morbidity disproportionately affects minority and low-income pregnant women, especially non-Hispanic Black women and those with Medicaid coverage.

Fingar KF (IBM Watson Health), Hambrick MM (AHRQ), Heslin KC (AHRQ), Moore JE (Institute for Medicaid Innovation). Trends and Disparities in Delivery Hospitalizations Involving Severe Maternal Morbidity, 2006-2015. HCUP Statistical Brief #243. September 2018.

Agency for Healthcare Research and Quality, Rockville, MD. www.hcup-us.ahrq.gov/reports/statbriefs/sb243-Severe-Maternal-Morbidity-Delivery-Trends-Disparities.pdf.

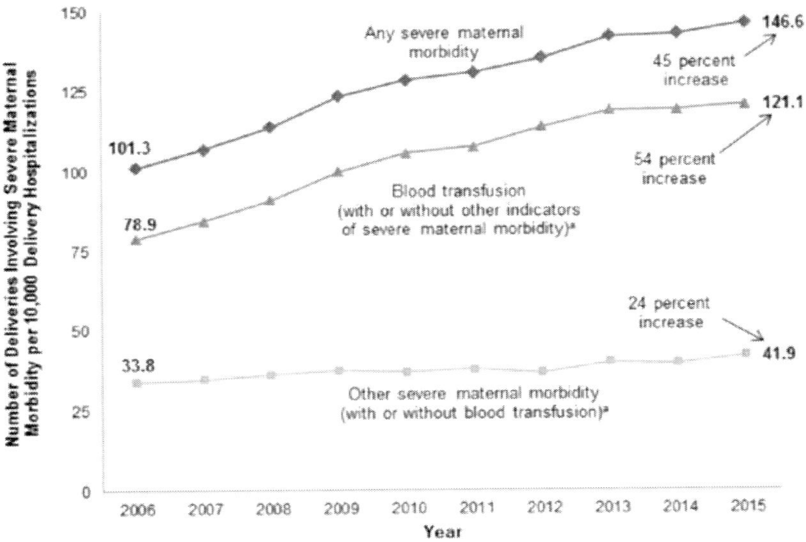

Figure 1. Trends in delivery hospitalizations involving severe maternal morbidity, 2005-2015.

The next graph depicts maternal death. American women are more than three times as likely to die in the maternal period and six times as likely to die as Scandinavians. In every other high-income country, many less affluent than the US, maternal mortality rates have been falling. But in the US, maternal deaths increased from 2000-2005, with the CDC estimating nearly 60% of such deaths are preventable.

Going forward we envision a society where every person can start or grow their family with dignity by accessing childbirth care that is safe, supportive and empowering. In the current state, maternal health is dangerously fragmented and riddled with inequity. The quality of care for women and moms can swing wildly from one woman to the next based on the accident of her geography, the color of her skin, or the size of her paycheck. Families, healthcare providers and policy makers must come together to shed light on where we are failing and how we can do better.

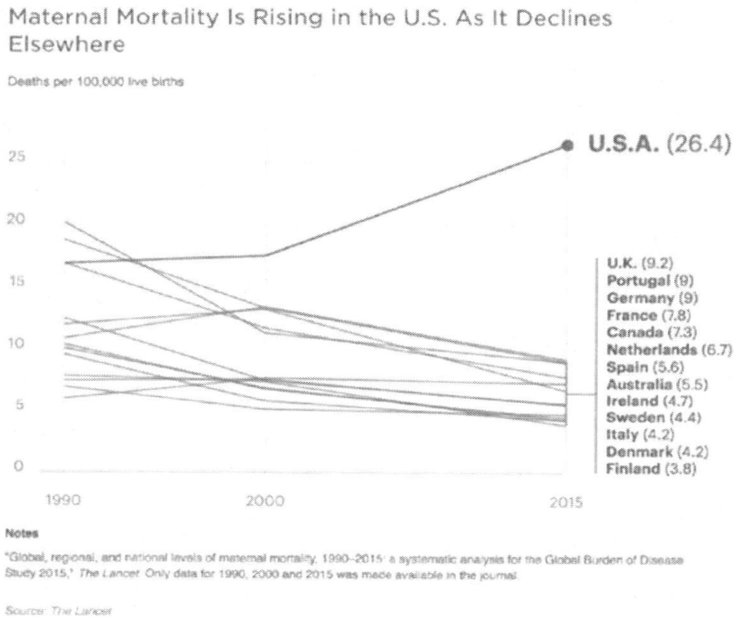

Figure 2.

We are pleased H.R. 1318 enjoys bipartisan support in the House and Senate. We applaud the Senate HELP Committee for advancing S. 1112, the Maternal Health Accountability Act this past June, and for taking a significant step toward fighting maternal mortality and improving maternal health. This legislation will help reverse our country's rising maternal mortality rate by assisting states to establish or improve multidisciplinary committees that will track, analyze and identify local solutions to prevent maternal deaths. These are known as maternal mortality review committees (MMRCs). And we are also pleased they raised the funding level available for these state MMRCs from $ 7 million to $12 million each year for five years. This increased investment will allow the CDC to robustly support state MMRCs so they can provide a comprehensive picture of why these deaths are occurring, and come up with actionable solutions.

Advancement of H.R. 1318 today shows House leadership in addressing this public health crisis, a first step in ending preventable maternal mortality.

Thank you for your consideration of this legislation on September 14th, 2018. We urge this Subcommittee and House to pass without delay. Feel free to contact either of us with any questions.

Respectfully,

Ginger Breedlove, PhD, CNM, FACNM
President, March for Moms
maternitycaremarch@gmail.com

Dr. Neel Shah, MD, MPP, FACOG
Vice-President, March for Moms

September 12, 2018

House of Representatives
Committee on Energy and Commerce
Washington DC

Dear Members of the Committee,

Having a new baby is supposed to be the happiest time in a woman's life. Not always.

New mothers in the United States are dying at increasing numbers. In fact, the United States has the highest rate of maternal mortality than any other developed country, and this rate continues to rise in our country as it declines elsewhere around the globe.

What is going on in the United States? Why are at least 700 new mothers dying each year?

Why has the rate of maternal mortality in the United States DOUBLED since 2000?

The only way to answer these questions is to review each and every maternal death through statewide maternal mortality review committees

(MMRCs), groups of maternal-child health experts and advocates who identify, review, and analyze maternal deaths and then disseminate information and act on the findings. Unfortunately, not all states have MMRCs, nor do the existing MMRCs gather data uniformly and consistently.

One of the leading causes of death for women in the first year after having a baby is SUICIDE. The United Kingdom and Japan both report suicide as the LEADING CAUSE of maternal mortality. Because we don't track this information in the United States, we are not sure of the suicide rate. But we know that postpartum depression and related mental health issues affect at least 1 in 5 women during pregnancy or first year postpartum. And we know that women like Shelane Gaydos, Allison Goldstein, and Brittany Butts (see next page for more about each of these lovely young mothers) are taking their lives. We need better systems to help these women and to identify why and how new mothers are dying.

Please vote for full funding of maternal mortality review committees in all 50 states.

Why? Because children need their mothers.

Sincerely,

Adrienne Griffen; Founder and Executive Director

SAMPLE - MATERNAL DEATHS BY SUICIDE

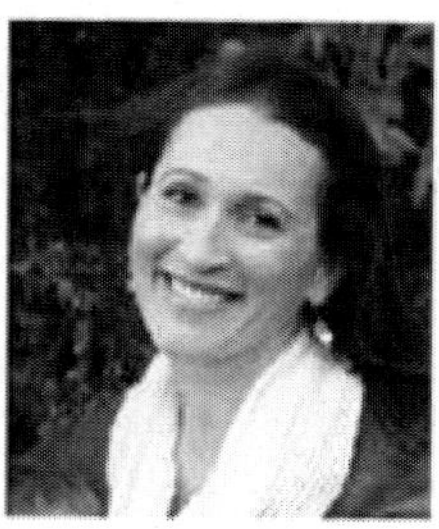

Shelane Dawn Gaydos

6/12/2015

Shelane was a strong, energetic, intelligent and warm woman. She had a hearty, infectious laugh and a bright smile. She was a loving and supportive wife to her husband, Brian, and a devoted mother to her three beautiful daughters, Nadia (7), Sofia (5) and Olivia (2). She truly lived for her girls and dedicated a lot of time and energy into making their lives extra special. On that beautiful sunny afternoon, after she made sure all the girls were safely at home and comfortable watching the T.V. she made an irreversible split minute decision to go into the next room, close the door and end her life.

Shelane was a Fairfax County police officer. Her family launched Shelane's Run 5K and Kids Fun Run in 2016 to raise awareness about PMADs. Learn more at www.shelanesrun.org.

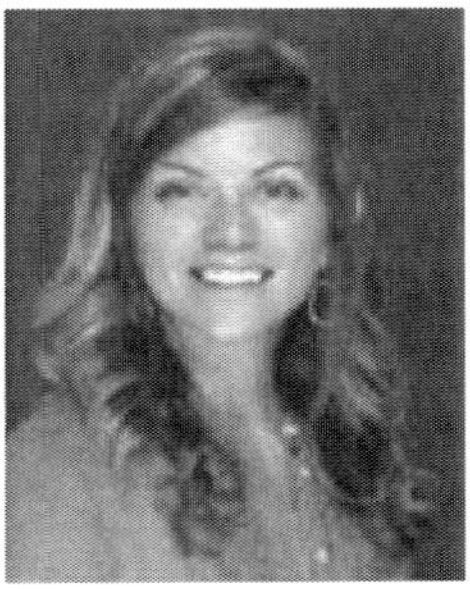

Allison Mathews Goldstein
6/28/2016

No star shone brighter, no smile was sweeter than Allison Goldstein. She was a wonderful Mother, a devoted wife, and remarkable daughter and sister, a special aunt to two nephews and a niece, five cousins and countless friends. Amidst all the joy and love she shared with the world, Allison silently suffered from postpartum depression. Allison is survived by her loving husband, Maj. Justin Goldstein, and her infant daughter, Ainslee Parker.

Allison's family has taken on the issue of maternal suicide through a foundation they launched named Allison's Reach and by speaking publicly and openly about their loss.

Allison's story has been featured in local news outlets and shared worldwide via social media.

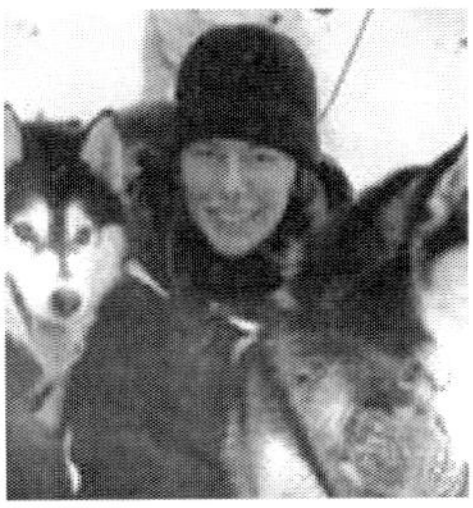

Brittany Julianna Butt
11/12/2014

Brittany loved being on the sled running with her Siberian Huskies, or showing them in the conformation ring. Mother to her son Teige, with husband Jeff, she was aspiring to be a sports veterinarian. Brittany was the spark in the room that made lasting impressions with everyone. She was loved by her family and friends. Yet none of us really knew the depth of her despair or the many questions that would be left unanswered.

Brittany's mother, Natalie Velasquez, participated in PMAD Advocacy Day in 2016. Natalie is a psychiatrist who lived in Northern Virginia for many years and now lives in Alaska

House Energy & Commerce Committee Health Subcommittee Hearing on Better Data and Better Outcomes: Reducing Maternal Mortality in the U.S., September 27, 2018, Testimony for the Record, Submitted by Susan Chacon, MSW, LISW, President, Association of Maternal & Child Health Programs (AMCHP)

Chairman Burgess, Ranking Member Green and distinguished members of the subcommittee, thank you for this opportunity to submit testimony in support of H.R. 1318, the Preventing Maternal Deaths Act. I would also like to especially thank Representatives Jaime Herrera Beutler

(R-WA) and Diana DeGette (D-CO) as well as their staff for their diligent work to introduce and refine this bill.

My name is Susan Chacon and I currently serve as the President of the Board of the Association of Maternal & Child Health Programs (AMCHP). For 16 years, AMCHP has collaborated with national partners to build the capacity of state- and jurisdiction-based teams to conduct maternal mortality and morbidity surveillance, including establishing and sustaining maternal mortality review committees. As an organization representing state maternal and child public health leaders, many of our members directly oversee the maternal mortality review committee process in their own states.

I am proud that my state of New Mexico, where I currently serve as the Children and Youth with Special Health Care Needs Director, has been conducting maternal mortality review in some form since 1980 and by a multidisciplinary committee since 1993. The mission of our maternal mortality review committee is to identify and review maternal deaths caused by pregnancy complications and other factors, to identify remediable problems contributing to maternal deaths, and to develop interventions to reduce these deaths.

This process is time consuming and resource intensive. Currently there is no dedicated federal source of funding for maternal mortality review committees and therefore most states cobble together funding from a combination of their Title V Maternal and Child Health Services Block Grant, fluctuating state funding allotments, private grants and volunteered time. Today, only 35 states (as well as 3 large cities) have maternal mortality review committees, which means they have the capacity to understand why mothers are dying and what can be done to prevent these tragedies. This capacity is fragile and easily influenced by shifting state public health priorities and funding constraints and must be nurtured to ensure adherence to best practices. The remaining one-third of states are in varying stages of forming a maternal mortality review committee and may be struggling in building political and social will or finding adequate funding and staff support to put a review committee into practice. Because these committees operate independently of one another and are governed by individual state laws and/or regulations, they are also vulnerable to inconsistent methods of collecting, analyzing, and reporting data, thereby hindering our ability to tell a complete national story about maternal mortality in the U.S.

H.R. 1318 would take a critical step forward by providing federal support to build and sustain the work of state maternal mortality review committees and advance efforts to standardize the review process and the collection and analysis of data. With this support, we can continue to work together to turn that data into action in order to save women's lives.

About AMCHP

The Association of Maternal & Child Health Programs is a national resource, partner and advocate for state public health leaders and others working to improve the health of women, children, youth and families, including those with special health care needs.

Heart Safe Motherhood at Penn Medicine (University of Pennsylvania Health System)

Website: https://healthcareinnovation.upenn.edu/projects/heart-safe-motherhood

Preeclampsia is a disorder of pregnancy characterized by high blood pressure and high levels of protein in the urine. Hypertension is the leading cause of maternal morbidity and mortality in the U.S., and while risk factors are known, previously no strategy existed for effective, reliable blood pressure surveillance for at-risk patients. With poor maternal outcomes on the rise in Philadelphia and across the country and new guidelines on postpartum care issued by the American College of Obstetricians and Gynecologists this spring, there is a clear call to action and an audience eager for a solution.

A Penn Medicine team, led by providers and researchers in Maternal Fetal Medicine, has designed a common-sense approach to care that answers an important challenge. Their solution, Heart Safe Motherhood (HSM), is an evidence-based care model with real-world data that's bolstering the promise of connected health, and by its focus on convenient care for women, speaks to the growing attention being paid to women as a vital demographic in the dual eras of population health and health care consumerism.

At the start of the HSM project, blood pressure monitoring required patients to attend a one-time, in-person appointment. However, professional association guidelines published by ACOG in 2014 recommended two points of monitoring: 72 hours and seven to ten days post-discharge.

As part of the project, the team developed and tested a text-based intervention for hypertension. They enrolled patients in a remote blood pressure monitoring program during the first seven days post-discharge from the Labor and Delivery floor at HUP.

Over the course of seven iterative pilots, over 30 patients were discharged with digital blood pressure monitors and sent reminders via text message to check their blood pressure twice daily. Once submitted by the patient, blood pressure results were reviewed and responded to by an Ob/Gyn physician.

After the conclusion of the pilot, the team received funding from the Penn PCORI Grant and Penn Presbyterian Harrison Fund to conduct a randomized controlled trial of the intervention. The team was recognized for their leadership with a first prize award in the American Heart Association's Philadelphia Heart Science Forum Innovation Challenge, Digital Health Category, and first place in the Council on Patient Safety in Women's Health National Improvement Challenge on Hypertension in Pregnancy.

Heart Safe Motherhood continues to make postpartum remote blood pressure monitoring easy so that providers can catch rising blood pressure earlier and keep patients safe at home.

Our journey to spread Heart Safe Motherhood has just begun. Heart Safe Motherhood can become a national model for reducing the burden of preeclampsia on maternal morbidity and mortality. Through text message-based remote monitoring, we have transformed our ability at one hospital to provide high quality, convenient, and safe care for women with pregnancy-related hypertension in the immediate postpartum period. We have developed knowledge about how to identify and enroll patients for engagement and how to capture and act on blood pressure remotely for clinical impact, providing the right care to the right patient at the right time. We have learned to think outside conventional medicine and listen to our patients. In fact, the American College of Obstetrics and Gynecology recently acknowledged our work in their May, 2018 Committee Opinion on Redefining the postpartum visit.

Through Heart Safe Motherhood, we can transform our ability to monitor hypertension remotely. The Heart Safe Motherhood program allows us to provide patient-centered postpartum care for women with preeclampsia who are at risk of devastating complications while simultaneously engaging them in their future health.

Program Results

Nine months ago, the team implemented Heart Safe Motherhood for patients with known pregnancy-related hypertension at the Hospital of the University of Pennsylvania. Since then, they have been able to obtain blood pressures remotely at the two time points recommended by ACOG in 80 percent of patients, intervene and start medications from home before development of morbidity, and continue to have strong patient and provider satisfaction. The team's readmission rate has dropped from 5 percent for postpartum patients monitored for hypertensive issues prior to Heart Safe Motherhood to 1 percent with the program at scale. Hypertension is no longer the leading cause of seven-day obstetrical readmissions at the Hospital of the University of Pennsylvania.

Additional proof points and tangible results include:

- Results of the pilot program showed there were no seven-day readmissions among enrolled patients, compared to a 5 percent readmission rate among women monitored through in-person visits. The percent of patients to report at least one blood pressure reading in the first week post-discharge jumped from 15 percent pre-intervention to 84 percent among all enrolled patients.
- The percent of patients to report blood pressure readings on five of seven days in the first week post-discharge jumped from 0 percent pre-intervention to 69 percent among all enrolled patients.
- At the conclusion of the RCT, the team saw the platform's ability to meet ACOG guidelines on postpartum blood monitoring leap from 0 percent to 82 percent compared to in-person office visits and seven-day readmissions from hypertension drop from 3 percent to 0 percent.

Heart Safe Motherhood is now the standard of care for obstetrics patients at HUP with plans to scale to other Penn Medicine locations in 2018. The team is also partnering with health systems, payers, and vendors to evaluate the ability to scale the program for national impact.

September 27, 2018

The Honorable Greg Walden
Chairman
Committee on Energy & Commerce U.S.
House of Representatives
Washington, DC

The Honorable Michael Burgess
Chairman
Subcommittee on Health
Committee on Energy & Commerce
U.S. House of Representatives
Washington, DC

The Honorable Frank Pallone
Ranking Member
Committee on Energy & Commerce
U.S. House of Representatives
Washington DC

The Honorable Gene Green
Ranking Member
Subcommittee on Health
Committee on Energy & Commerce
U.S. House of Representatives
Washington DC

Dear Chairman Walden, Ranking Member Pallone, Chairman Burgess and Ranking Member Green:

Our organizations commend you for holding today's hearing, "Better Data and Better Outcomes: Reducing Maternal Mortality in the U.S." We would like to express our support for the discussion draft of H.R. 1318, the Preventing Maternal Deaths Act, sponsored by Representatives Jaime Herrera Beutler (R-WA), Diana DeGette (D-CO) and Ryan Costello (R-PA) that is being considered today, which mirrors S. 1112, the Maternal Health Accountability Act, as recently advanced by the Senate HELP Committee.

Our nation faces a growing crisis in maternal health. More women die from pregnancy-related complications in the United States than in any other developed country, and the rate of maternal deaths continues to rise. Major disparities in maternal mortality exist, with black women three to four times more likely than white women to die during pregnancy or shortly after birth. Moreover, for every maternal death that occurs, an estimated 100 other women suffer severe complications of pregnancy or childbirth. We must act now to reverse this trend and save mothers' lives.

We urge the Subcommittee to address maternal mortality by supporting the work of state maternal mortality review committees (MMRCs) through the Centers for Disease Control and Prevention (CDC).

MMRCs are multidisciplinary groups of local experts in maternal, infant, and public health that examine cases of maternal death. Maternal mortality review is a cyclical process that does not end by simply counting and characterizing deaths, but must be followed with action by putting the recommendations of the committee to work in hospitals, communities, or policies.

While these efforts take place at the state or jurisdiction level, federal support will accelerate progress toward ensuring that every state has a high-functioning MMRC. This legislation will also advance efforts among states to standardize the collection and analysis of data. With better data and information, we can develop a national understanding of why mothers are dying and what we collectively can do to reverse this tragic trend.

We look forward to continuing to work together to see this bipartisan bill move forward in Congress and enacted into law.

Sincerely,

1,000 Days
2020 Mom
AFE Foundation
American Academy of Family Physicians
American Academy of Pediatrics
American College of Nurse-Midwives
American College of Obstetricians and Gynecologists
American College of Physicians
American College of Surgeons
American Medical Women's Association
American Psychological Association
American Public Health Association
American Society for Reproductive Medicine
Amnesty International USA
APS Foundation of America, Inc.
Association for Prevention Teaching and Research
Association of Maternal & Child Health Programs
Association of Public Health Laboratories

Association of Schools and Programs of Public Health

Association of State and Territorial Health Officials

Association of State Public Health Nutritionists (ASPHN) MCH Nutrition Council

Association of Women's Health, Obstetric and Neonatal Nurses

Children's Defense Fund

Choices in Childbirth

Every Child by Two

Every Mother Counts

Genetic Alliance

Hand to Hold

HER Foundation

Heroes for Moms

Lamaze International

March of Dimes

Maternal Safety Foundation

Medicines360

MomsRising

NAPHSIS

National Association of County and City Health Officials

National Association of Nurse Practitioners in Women's Health

National Association of Pediatric Nurse Practitioners

National Association of Perinatal Social Workers

National Black Women's HIV/AIDS Network

National Blood Clot Alliance

National Health Law Program

National Partnership for Women & Families

National Perinatal Association

National WIC Association

New York State Birth Center Association

Nurse-Family Partnership

Organization of Teratology Information Specialists

Patient Safety Movement Foundation

PCOS Challenge: The National Polycystic Ovary Syndrome Association

Power to Decide, the campaign to prevent unplanned pregnancy

Preeclampsia Foundation

Preemie World, LLC

Safe States Alliance

Save the Mommies Inc.

Society for Maternal Fetal Medicine

Society for Public Health Education

Spina Bifida Association

The 2 Degrees Foundation

The National Accreta Foundation

The National Alliance to Advance Adolescent Health

The Shane Foundation

The Tara Hansen Foundation

The Tatia Oden French Memorial Foundation

Trust for America's Health

United Methodist Women

ZERO TO THREE

Written Testimony of Catherine Glenn Foster President and CEO, Americans United for Life Regarding the Subcommittee Hearing, Better Data and Better Outcomes: Reducing Maternal Mortality in the U.S. Submitted to the House Energy and Commerce Subcommittee on Health Thursday, September 27, 2018

Chairman Burgess, Ranking Member Green, and distinguished Members of the Committee:

Americans United for Life (AUL) urges the Committee to recognize that not all maternal mortality is the same and to include specific statistical data collection and reporting on abortion-related mortality in the Preventing Maternal Deaths Act of 2018. Founded in 1971, Americans United for Life, the legal architect of the prolife movement, is a national law and policy nonprofit organization with a specialization in abortion and bioethics law.

The current United States system for reporting abortion-related maternal mortality is deeply flawed, and there is currently no reliable source of data. For the sake of women's health, this Committee should take steps to remedy that problem.

Abortion data reporting in the U.S. is entirely voluntary. This skews both the statistics and resulting analysis. For the reporting that does occur, maternal mortality due to abortion is often underreported as many maternal deaths are attributed to some other cause—like "sepsis," or "infection"—rather than the true underlying cause, termination of the pregnancy. This means that most studies are based on abortion "estimates" and "reported" deaths.[25] Additional studies show that 1 out of 16 women who have an abortion will visit an emergency room within six weeks after the abortion,[26] which, due to data collection methodology, should be considered a floor and not a ceiling.

Abortion-related maternal deaths are not systemically collected. There are two national reporting organizations: the Alan Guttmacher Institute (AGI) and the Centers for Disease Control and Prevention (CDC). AGI collects its data from abortion providers that report voluntarily. The CDC collects its data from the states, which report data haphazardly. For example, California— where reportedly one-third to one-half of all abortions in the U.S. are performed—has not reported its data to the CDC for several years. The numbers of annual abortions reported by AGI and the CDC differ by 15% or more.

---

[25] *See, e.g.*, Elizabeth G. Raymond & David A. Grimes, *The Comparative Safety of Legal Induced Abortion and Childbirth in the United States*, 119 Obstetrics & Gynecology 215 (2012).

[26] Ushma D. Upadhyay et al., *Incidence of Emergency Department Visits and Complications After Abortion*, 125 Obstetrics & Gynecology 175, 175 (2015).

The deeply flawed state of abortion-related maternal health data collection and reporting is a direct risk to the health of women. It deprives doctors of accurate data, which in turn prevents them from providing accurate information about abortion-related maternal mortality and morbidity to women. This is even more problematic considering the vast majority of abortions are elective and not medically indicated.

With the current data and reporting regime, it is impossible for a woman considering undergoing an abortion to receive the information she needs to voluntarily consent. Women need more than "estimates" or "guesses" on abortion-related maternal mortality to make an informed decision. They need complete and accurate data, and the U.S. has a responsibility to care for women's health by providing this data through public health reports.

Such a dysfunctional system of abortion-related maternal health data collection and reporting in the U.S. is unnecessarily substandard. In contrast, the collection and reporting of births and other gynecological procedures in the U.S. is systematic and thorough. Unlike maternal mortality from natural causes, abortion-related maternal mortality can be directly linked to either an invasive surgical procedure or a chemically-induced response. Given that this unnatural impact to pregnancy is man-made, it stands to reason that there should exist a robust methodology to track its impact. Currently, there is not.

In conclusion, this Committee should add data collection and reporting on abortion-related maternal mortality specifically in the Preventing Maternal Deaths Act of 2018.

Sincerely,

Catherine Glenn Foster, MA, JD
President and CEO
Americans United for Life

Nurse-Family Partnership
Helping First-Time Parents Succeed

1900 Grant Street, 4th Floor / Denver CO 80203 / 866.864.5226 / nursefamilypartnership.org

September 26, 2018

The Honorable Michael Burgess
United States House of Representatives
Washington D.C. 20515

Dear Chairman Burgess,

As a board member of Nurse-Family Partnership (NFP), I write in strong support of H.R. 1318, the *Preventing Maternal Deaths Act of 2017*. NFP is an evidence-based community health program with a core mission of improving the lives of at-risk moms and their children, and we thank you for your attention and steadfast commitment to improving maternal health outcomes.

Each day, NFP nurses work in their local communities to transform the lives of at-risk, first-time mothers. The program partners mothers with a registered nurse at a pivotal moment — beginning early in pregnancy with a first child – and provides ongoing nurse home visits that continue through her child's second birthday. Their relationship begins with a focus on the mother – their personal goals as well as their overall health -- which leads to healthier outcomes in both the mother and child after birth. Specifically, a 20-year follow-up study of an NFP randomized controlled trial in Memphis, TN found that NFP is effective at reducing all-cause mortality among mothers and preventable-cause mortality in their first-born children living in highly disadvantaged settings. This study showed that mothers who did not receive nurse home-visits were nearly 3 times more likely to die from all causes of death than nurse-visited moms.

We believe that H.R. 1318 stands to greatly improve how we address maternal mortality in this country, by providing needed federal support for Maternal Mortality Review Committees (MMRCs). These committees bring together stakeholders to focus on locally-relevant, preventative solutions that work and investing in those that are effective, like NFP.

We are so grateful for your continued leadership on this critical issue. Please let us know if we can be a resource to you as you work to advance this legislation.

Sincerely,

Fred Cerise
CEO, Parkland Health & Hospital System

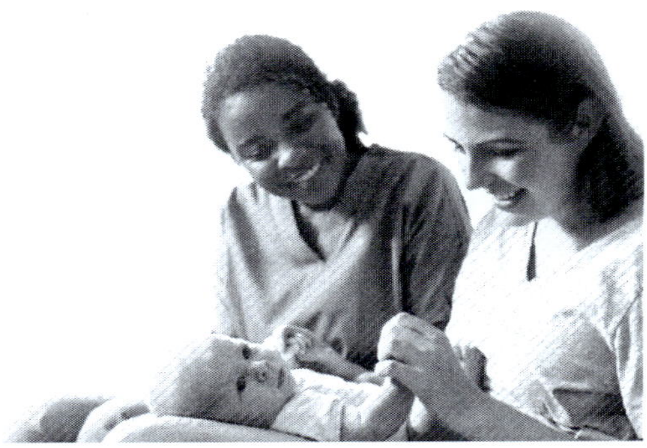

House Energy & Commerce Committee Health Subcommittee Hearing on "Better Data and Better Outcomes: Reducing Maternal Mortality in the U.S.," September 27, 2018, Testimony for the Record, Submitted by Eleni Tsigas, Chief Executive Officer, Preeclampsia Foundation

Chairman Burgess, Ranking Member Green, and distinguished members of the subcommittee, thank you for holding today's hearing to address "Better Data and Better Outcomes: Reducing Maternal Mortality in the U.S." I am Eleni Tsigas, Chief Executive Officer of the Preeclampsia Foundation, and I am so pleased for the opportunity to submit testimony for this hearing in support of the discussion draft of H.R. 1318, the *Preventing Maternal Deaths Act*. I would also like to recognize the hard work of Representatives Jaime Herrera Beutler (R-WA) and Diana DeGette (D-CO) for their efforts to address the crisis of maternal mortality in the U.S. and to introduce and advance this important legislation.

Preeclampsia is one of the leading causes of mothers dying from pregnancy-related issues. It is a hypertensive disorder of pregnancy characterized by high blood pressure, protein in the urine, and sometimes failure of the kidneys, liver and other organs. It can affect up to one in 12 pregnancies, and there is no cure, only management.

Nineteen years ago, I held the still warm body of my baby daughter in my arms and kissed her desperately, trying to will her back to life. My kidneys had failed. I had lost half of my body's blood volume when I delivered her because of an undetected placental abruption due to preeclampsia, and I almost died. So many other women like me have faced similar circumstances, but sadly, many of them did not survive and cannot offer their testimony here today.

As an organization, the Preeclampsia Foundation is focused on educating patients, their families and health care providers to recognize the preeclampsia warning signs and ensure that timely care is provided so no woman dies during pregnancy, delivery, or during the postpartum period. Moving this agenda forward has required solid data proving that a lack of patient knowledge of preeclampsia is a factor in a large percentage of preventable deaths. We have been able to obtain much of this data from existing state maternal mortality review committees, but much more data is needed. The data from state maternal mortality review committees is utilized to ensure healthcare providers accept and adopt the Preeclampsia Foundation's call to action to educate women about the signs and symptoms of preeclampsia and appropriately respond with timely diagnosis and accurate clinical management when they do.

Thanks to the work of existing maternal mortality review committees, the Foundation is sending out hundreds of thousands of pieces of patient education materials every year that are used in hospitals, and often in prenatal care settings. We strive to push out millions of educational materials, and women should be getting them at every prenatal visit, but unfortunately, too many states have not yet been able to - or understood how to - appropriately collect and assess their maternal mortality data that is linked to hypertensive disorders of pregnancy or other pregnancy-related complications.

The Preeclampsia Foundation ultimately strives to prevent maternal mortality and severe maternal morbidity and help states and communities establish protocols that save lives. We view this as a data-to-action initiative. There is so much to be learned from maternal mortality reviews that can improve healthcare practices today. For example, in Florida, based on their maternal mortality reviews, the state found that hospitals were taking too long to treat pregnant women that had severe high blood pressure. These women were dying from stroke and other preventable sequelae. Armed with data, new standards and protocols were set. In less than a year, 90 percent of women with persistent new onset severe hypertension were treated within one hour in hospitals using a new hypertension in pregnancy protocol. Before that time, only 20 percent were being treated within one hour.

Another example of where data can impact care is in addressing postpartum preeclampsia. One of the most common myths associated with this disorder is that "delivery is the cure for preeclampsia." This is not true. Women are still at risk from preeclampsia and related hypertensive disorders following delivery, sometimes for weeks, particularly as most care is directed to the baby. Analyses from some states' data has reinforced this by reviewing the number of mothers that die after they have returned home post delivery. We need far better postpartum surveillance, and we need to train emergency departments for when these women present with signs of preeclampsia-related distress. We cannot let up after delivery. There are states to learn from that have successfully begun to address postpartum preeclampsia. The legislation the Committee is reviewing here today would do much to support this type of information exchange to share best practices with other states.

Preeclampsia costs the U.S. health care system $2.18 billion dollars a year – about half due to maternal health care costs and half for the care of the infants born to those mothers. To put that into perspective, these preeclampsia-related costs comprise about 1/3 of the costs for these entire pregnancies in just one year. The long-term costs associated with prematurity and long-term maternal health consequences are not included in these numbers.

A long time health activist, Mary Lasker, once said, "Research is expensive, but disease is more!" In the case of maternal mortality reviews, the research that is collected, assessed, and released by the state committees almost immediately leads to health care improvements and is nowhere near as expensive as the health conditions and complexities we would otherwise face. There are system factors, patient factors and provider factors that contribute to maternal mortality and severe morbidity today. We can do so much more with a small investment of time and resources for states and ultimately improve outcomes for thousands of lives. This must be a public health priority. Maternal health is the building block upon which all other health issues are based. We need compelling, instructive data to move healthcare providers and institutions to action and to support patient and family engagement in their health care.

Support the H.R. 1318 Discussion Draft

Mr. Chairman, Ranking Member Green and members of the Subcommittee, the discussion draft of H.R. 1318, *The Preventing Maternal Deaths Act*, sponsored by Representatives Jaime Herrera Beutler (R-WA), Diana DeGette (D-CO), and Ryan Costello (R-PA) mirrors S. 1112, the *Maternal Health Accountability Act*, as recently passed by the Senate Committee on Health, Education, Labor and Pensions.

This legislation will help support state efforts to get at solutions – affordable and actionable efforts that can save lives. The bill, with the support and expertise of the Centers for Disease Control and Prevention (CDC) will help states understand how to identify local problems that contribute to rising rates of maternal mortality and derive local solutions. It will also help states that have been unable to get a maternal mortality review committee launched or operating. Despite the pockets of successful committees, the fact remains that today no state has a fully functioning maternal mortality review committee; even the best of them are handicapped by inadequate information, resources or know-how. For too many, the investment that has been made to date in databases, training, and tools will have been wasted if we cannot create a sustainable maternal mortality review system and thereby demonstrate what we value most: our mothers.

The Preeclampsia Foundation believes the discussion draft of H.R. 1318 will work to put an end to the rising rate of maternal mortality in the United States, protecting our mothers and saving health care resources. On behalf of the Foundation and all of the families we represent, we urge the Committee to prioritize this legislation and for Congress to pass it this year.

SEPTEMBER 24, 2018, STATEMENT OF TIMORIA MCQUEEN SABA, SURVIVOR OF A NEAR FATAL POSTPARTUM HEMORRHAGE, COMMISSIONER FOR THE COMMONWEALTH OF MASSACHUSETTS, SENATOR ELLEN STORY SPECIAL COMMISSION ON POSTPARTUM DEPRESSION, BEFORE THE SUBCOMMITTEE ON HEALTH COMMITTEE ON ENERGY AND COMMERCE U.S. HOUSE OF REPRESENTATIVES, "BETTER DATA AND BETTER OUTCOMES: REDUCING MATERNAL MORTALITY IN THE U.S."

Dear Mr. Chairman, Ranking Member Green, members of the committee: My name is Timoria McQueen Saba.

I am an African-American mother of two daughters, Graison Joyce and Harper Elle. I've waited many years to see a bill like this get passed. On April 19, 2010, I started hemorrhaging after giving birth to Graison. My uterus wouldn't contract after the birth, known as a uterine atony. Doctors told me that they would try to save my uterus and ovaries by performing a procedure called an embolization. If that was not successful, they would have to give me a hysterectomy. If the bleeding continued after receiving a hysterectomy, I was told that I would die.

My pregnancy with Graison can best be described as "normal." I had no pre-existing conditions and am fortunate to have great health insurance. I had a relatively easy, but long (twenty-seven hour) labor. Once I was fully dilated, delivery was fast and easy — I remember thinking it was almost *too* easy. Ten pushes and twenty minutes later, my beautiful daughter was born. As I held Graison in my arms for a few moments, I could feel a shift in the mood of the hospital staff in the room. Before I knew it, the serenity of the room was tainted by the sounds of warning beeps from the machines I was hooked up to. Next, the room became flooded with strangers.

Enter emergency personnel. My husband, Robert, and Graison were rushed out of the room and taken into the nursery. I watched blood pour out of my vagina through the reflection from an overhead television screen. My body was weak, and I struggled to keep my eyes open, feeling deep down that if I allowed them to close they would never open again. After a three-hour long surgery (during which I was fully conscious), I was left in critical condition. Instead of staying in intensive care alone, my Ob/Gyn insisted that I be reunited with Graison and Robert in the labor and delivery ward.

I was told not to move a muscle, which included nursing or holding my new baby. I lay awake all night in pain. I was afraid to sleep, afraid to move, afraid that every breath I took might shake loose whatever was keeping me together. I stared at Graison all night. Her big, round, brown eyes peered through the bassinet. I made a promise to her that I would be live — she would *not* be a motherless child. I survived and the three of us went home five days later.

I was diagnosed with PTSD (Post Traumatic Stress Disorder) several weeks after giving birth. Because of what happened, I was afraid to leave the house. This was a very new feeling to me. At the time, I was a professional make-up artist and loved traveling with my clients to destinations near and far. I had never been afraid to go anywhere! After the traumatic birth, I was easily startled and wrought with anxiety that something might happen to me, my daughter or my husband.

It became increasingly difficult to sleep at night. Every time I closed my eyes, I saw the blood pouring from my body and other reminders of the ordeal I had suffered through. Due to the demands of motherhood, I tried to push my negative feelings aside. I was excited to be a mom and savored the days I spent with Graison. I challenged myself to get out of the house. I joined a hospital support group for new moms and signed up for "Mommy and Me" baby music classes. As I met more new moms I felt a common bond among us as we talked about breastfeeding, sleep schedules and baby gear. We also shared intimate details of our lives that you would never think possible to share with strangers. I made great friends through joining that group. Despite my outgoing nature and positive outlook on life, deep inside I remained a traumatized victim of a near fatal postpartum hemorrhage. No other mom I met back then had experienced a postpartum hemorrhage. My feelings about the hemorrhage and the surgery never went away. My emotions cycled through anger, guilt, fear and sadness.

Thirteen months after Graison was born, I had a miscarriage which resulted in another hemorrhage. This occurred in front of several people while I was in a frozen yogurt shop. The miscarriage triggered the difficult emotions from the hemorrhage I suffered the year prior. I underwent an emergency D &C and returned home the next day. Yet again- I was sad, angry and afraid that I might bleed to death at any moment.

I knew that I could not be the *only* woman who experienced these types of harrowing birth and pregnancy complications. While looking for answers, I realized that resources and support for mothers and families who had survived a near miss or lost a loved one due to a birth or pregnancy complication, were scarce. I began sharing my story publicly in 2012 and have since connected with thousands of women across America who have experienced similar birth and pregnancy complications; and the lingering psychological effects. With the help of a therapist who specializes in postpartum mental health and birth trauma, I was able to heal. I gave birth to Harper Elle in March 2014. I'm happy to report that my birth experience the second time around was perfectly "normal."

I am now a full-time maternal health advocate, speaker and writer with a focus on mental and physical trauma due to childbirth and pregnancy. I am also the coordinator of resources and support for Postpartum Support International (PSI) in the Boston Metro West and Central areas. In this role, I connect women suffering from postpartum mood disorders and their families to local therapists and support groups. I'm also a member of the PSI President's Advisory Council. Twice per month, I facilitate a free peer-to-peer mother's support group, *Emotional Wellbeing After Baby*, at Milford Regional Hospital in Milford, MA. In 2017, I was honored to be appointed by MA State Rep. James O'Day (D-14 Worcester) to a House chair seat on the Senator Ellen Story Special Commission on Postpartum Depression.

Every day I think about how fortunate I am. I survived two hemorrhages due to birth and pregnancy complications. Statistics show that black mothers die during childbirth at three to four times the rate of white mothers.

Statistically speaking, I shouldn't be alive.

But because I survived, it is my duty and a privilege to be a voice for mothers who struggle to cope with the mental and physical effects of a near fatal birth trauma, and also honor those who tragically, have died.

Passing HR 1318: Preventing Maternal Mortality Act of 2017 is imperative to the health of all mothers and families in the United States. Individual states will be able to learn the exact causes of deaths due to childbirth and pregnancy complications, therefore helping healthcare providers to identify the proper preventions or the best emergency response plans.

It is our responsibility to care for *all* mothers in America. Legislators, healthcare providers, advocates and patients must work together to give mothers the healthcare they deserve. By passing this bill and working together to understand the disparities in outcomes, we will prevent mothers from dying and save entire generations from suffering.

Thank you for allowing me the opportunity to share my story with you.

June 27, 2018
The Honorable Jaime Herrera Beutler
U.S. House of Representatives
Washington DC

The Honorable Ryan Costello
U.S. House of Representatives
Washington, DC

The Honorable Diana DeGette
U.S. House of Representatives
Washington DC

Dear Representatives Herrera Beutler, Costello, and DeGette:

On behalf of the more than 80,000 members of the American College of Surgeons (ACS), I would like to express our support for the *Preventing Maternal Deaths Act*, H.R. 1318. This bipartisan legislation is an important step in addressing disparities in pregnancy-related mortality and identifying ways to make pregnancy safer.

The U.S. is the only industrialized nation with a rising maternal mortality rate. The U.S. saw a 26% increase in the maternal mortality rate from 18.8 deaths per 100,000 live births in 2000 to 23.8 in 2014.[27] Considerable racial disparities in pregnancy-related mortality exist. According to the Centers for Disease Control and Prevention's Pregnancy Mortality Surveillance System, during 2011–2013, the pregnancy-related mortality ratios were 12.7 deaths per 100,000 live births for white women compared to 43.5 deaths per 100,000 live births for black women.

According to the CDC Foundation, the leading causes of pregnancy-related death include seven causes accounting for 72.2% of all pregnancy-related deaths. The leading underlying causes of pregnancy-related death are hemorrhage, cardiovascular and coronary conditions, cardiomyopathy, infection, embolism, mental health conditions, and preeclampsia. Variations amongst the leading causes exist among states, race-ethnicity, and age. Determining methods to address disparities amongst different populations by providing high quality care will help to improve health outcomes.

Currently, 33 states are studying local maternal death cases through maternal mortality review committees (MMRCs) to identify opportunities for prevention and ways to make pregnancy safer for all women. The authorization of a Department of Health and Human Services (HHS) grant program through the Centers for Disease Control and Prevention (CDC) for states to establish, maintain, or expand MMRCs is critical for improving health outcomes and reducing disparities in pregnancy-related care.

---

[27] MacDorman, M., Declercq, E., Cabral, H., Morton, C., "Is the United States Maternal Mortality Rate Increasing? Disentangling trends from measurement issues: Short title: U.S. Maternal Mortality Trends." *Journal of Obstetrics and Gynecology*. September, 2016.

The ACS also strongly supports the provision directing HHS to research disparities in maternal health outcomes and expand access to health care services that improve quality and outcomes of maternity care for vulnerable populations. The establishment of a demonstration project to compare the effectiveness of and implement effective interventions to reduce disparities in maternity care is vital to efforts to reduce preventable pregnancy-related mortality.

Again, thank you for your leadership in introducing the *Preventing Maternal Deaths Act*. We look forward to working with you as this important legislation moves through Congress.

Sincerely,

David B. Hoyt, MD, FACS
Executive Director, American College of Surgeons
SAP America, Inc.
Washington DC

The Honorable Michael C. Burgess, MD
Chairman
Subcommittee on Health
Committee on Energy & Commerce
U.S. House of Representatives
Washington DC

The Honorable Gene Green
Ranking Member
Subcommittee on Health
Committee on Energy & Commerce
U.S. House of Representatives
Washington DC

September 28, 2018

RE: Submission Request for the Record of the Health Subcommittee's hearing entitled "Better Data and Better Outcomes: Reducing Maternal Mortality in the U.S.," being held on September 27, 2018

Dear Mr. Chairman and Ranking Member Green:

On behalf of SAP America Inc. (SAP), I write to respectfully request this letter and its accompanying attachments be entered into the Record of the Health Subcommittee's hearing entitled "Better Data and Better Outcomes: Reducing Maternal Mortality in the U.S.," being held on September 27, 2018.

SAP is the world's largest provider of enterprise application software serving over 400,000 customers and 100,00 partners in 180 countries. We develop and produce software for a wide range of customers, in both the public and private sectors, around the world. Seventy-seven percent of all global commercial transactions run through SAP software.

The extraordinary growth in the amounts of data available to governments presents both great challenges and significant opportunities. SAP has significant experience in translating those challenges to successful outcomes allowing governments to take advantage of the opportunities data and the analysis of the wealth of data at governments' fingertips present. Weaving together publicly held data sets holds great potential for making government more effective at serving the public.

In March 2014, then-Governor Pence of Indiana established the Indiana Management Performance Hub (MPH). Among the purposes of the MPH is to collect data from all Indiana state agencies and analyze the data to produce "continuous process improvements" by providing recommendations to the Governor on "[o]pportunities to use data . . . to drive innovation and efficiency . . . ." *See* Goldberg, "Analytics Paves the Way for Better Government," Forbes Insights, Sept. 2014, enclosed with this letter. SAP provides the software that performed the data analysis conducted by the MPH.

Of direct relevance to the Subcommittee's hearing on maternal mortality is the initial area of inquiry conducted in 2014 by the MPH. That initial study was focused on reducing infant mortality in Indiana. The report produced as a result of the study by KSM Consulting, entitled "A Summary of Findings and Quantitative Investigation Targeted at: Reducing Infant Mortality in Indiana," is attached for the Subcommittee's review and consideration, insofar as it may be relevant to the related subject of this hearing, the reduction in maternal mortality.

The Honorable Michael C. Burgess, MD
The Honorable Gene Green

September 27, 2018

As a result of the data analysis performed in connection with the MPH's review of infant mortality, Indiana was able to develop a set of predictive algorithms and put in place programs to address identify the most at-risk populations and ensure the delivery of services to this population by the Indiana State Department of Health.

SAP believes that programs like the Indiana MPH can and should be established at the state and local levels with federal support. The wider establishment of programs like the MPH can be a basis for the widespread improvement nationally on addressing maternal mortality rates.

The potential for emerging technologies to enable data-driven policy and practice is well articulated by the Commission on Evidence-based Policymaking: "…the Commission envisions a future in which rigorous evidence is created efficiently, as a routine part of government operations, and used to construct effective public policy. Advances in technology and statistical methodology, coupled with a modern legal framework and a commitment to transparency, make it possible to do this while simultaneously providing stronger protections for the privacy and confidentiality of the people, businesses, and organizations from which the government collects information. Addressing barriers to the use of already collected data is a path to unlocking important insights for addressing society's greatest challenges"[28]

SAP would be pleased to brief the Subcommittee members and staff on the MPH and the potential for data analytics in tackling many of government's most pressing problems.

Respectfully submitted,

Kevin M. Richards
Vice President, Head of US Government Relations
SAP America, Inc.

ANALYTICS PAVES THE WAY FOR BETTER GOVERNMENT

Forbes Insight
CASE STUDY

The State of Indiana is applying data-driven insights to improve outcomes for citizens and make public sector performance more transparent.

By Michael S. Goldberg

Managing state government often requires impassioned debate about the best way to allocate resources, deliver services to citizens and build budgets that reflect elected leaders' and citizens' priorities. The State of Indiana is bringing data-driven insights to these discussions through its use of analytics.

[28] Commission on Evidence-based Policymaking (https://www.cep.gov/content/dam/cep/report/cep-final-report.pdf).

Public sector organizations globally are fertile ground for policymakers' vision of more effective, timely decisions. Every agency, department and bureau has years' worth of data that has been collected in compliance with documented procedures, subject to oversight and accessible via information systems. Citizens, in fact, increasingly expect government agencies to manage and analyze their voluminous data sets in ways that benefit the public and enable government transparency.

Government leaders, from the European Commission to the White House, have called for investment in big data analytics capabilities to modernize government services and aid their economies. Deeper insights from government data offer more than the possibility for better-informed policy decisions. Businesses may also use these insights to create new data-driven products and services using government data (see Figure 1, "Data That Serves the Public"). In fact, McKinsey & Co. estimates that by digitizing information, disseminating public data sets and applying analytics to improve decision-making, governments around the world can act as catalysts for more than $3 trillion in economic value.[29]

In the State of Indiana, data is at the center of Gov. Mike Pence's long-term vision for improving the management and effectiveness of government programs and making Indiana a leader in data-driven decision-making. In March 2014, a year after taking office, Pence ordered state agencies to share data and partner with the state Office of Management and Budget (OMB, which oversees state finances and agency performance management), the Indiana Office of Technology (IOT) and outside experts in a centralized effort "to improve and strengthen services, maximize the utilization of available resources and ensure that state services are available to all." As in many public sector settings—where systems and tools have become available to more easily analyze large, diverse data sets—data sharing had not, until recently, been a common practice in states.

---

[29] Chui, Michael, Diana Farrell and Kate Jackson. "How Government Can Promote Open Data and Help Unleash Over $3 Trillion in Economic Value." McKinsey & Co., April 2014. http://goo.gl/Vusv99.

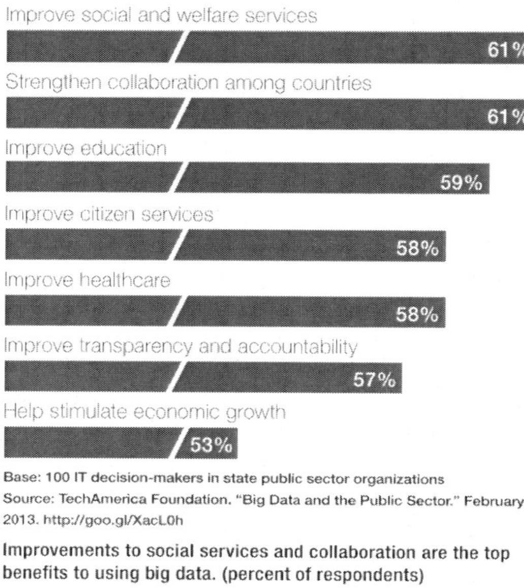

Figure 3. Data That Serves the Public.

Overseen by the OMB, the data-sharing mandate is setting the stage for an enterprise-wide solution that will put key performance indicators (KPIs) in front of decision-makers and the public. The solution will also apply both descriptive and predictive analytics to critical problems.

> By augmenting existing research efforts, analytics have the potential to uncover new approaches to stubborn problems.

Data Sharing Serves Policy Goals

Indiana's initiative aligns with the administration's six-pronged roadmap that emphasizes economic growth, education and the well-being of families (see Figure 2, "Data-Driven Progress"). "This project is enabling state government to service those goals and achieve outcomes," says OMB Director Chris Atkins.

Each of Indiana's 92 agencies and departments has a role to play. Using Gov. Pence's data-sharing order as a lever, Atkins and his colleagues are working with the IOT and the other agency heads to collect data for analysis. Part of Atkins' job is communicating the end-goal. "We're trying to help the agencies see the value in this project," he says. "A culture of data-sharing means a more successful enterprise."

Data sharing is more than a technical issue, as laws and regulations restrict the handling of certain types of data. So another essential element for Atkins was to hire several legal experts who could answer questions about the rules for using different data sets. Federal or state privacy laws may require agencies to remove personal information, for example. "We hired counsel to help the agencies work through these data security issues so they don't have to task their own legal teams," he says. "We're doing it for them, in concert with their leadership" (see Figure 3, "Breaking Down Barriers").

Analytics for Saving Lives

The data collection effort supports a four-point program to deliver more insights to government policymakers and the public. One segment, recently begun, targets a vital public policy problem: the rate of infant mortality in Indiana, which at 7.6 percent in 2010 ranked higher than the national average of 6.1 percent.

The project pilots Indiana's recently acquired in-memory computing platform, which supports predictive analytics capabilities. An in-memory platform enables organizations to consolidate extremely large volumes of data from multiple sources into one database and answers any question almost instantly. Indiana is now able to collect data sets from many different state agencies for rapid-fire, iterative queries. That ability, in turn, enables analysts to test out hypotheses and answer questions using a range of techniques and algorithms.

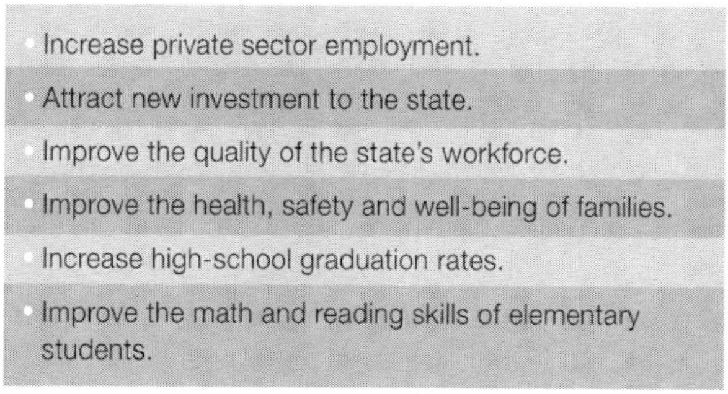

Figure 4. Data-Driven Progress.

By scrutinizing combinations of these data sources— and adding new data sources to the mix—analysts are working to identify correlations that provide signals about the possible causes of the infant mortality problem. The signals may relate to demographics, mothers' health conditions or unexpected relationships among other variables that influence babies' health.

The pilot so far is demonstrating the value of both the cooperation of state agencies (the shared data sets are useful in the predictive models) and the in-memory platform that provides fast response times to analysts' queries. Atkins says the work to date has shown promising results, but it's not finished. "We know as we add more data, we will see more results," he adds.

The findings are expected to drive the development of new programs or the updating of existing ones, so that the state can improve Indiana's performance—and reduce the number of infant deaths in Indiana. Charlie Brandt, managing director at KSM Consulting, a technology, management and data analytics consultancy that has been working with the state, says predictive analytics has the potential to elevate public policy decision-making as leaders are provided knowledge of drivers of transformation instead of reports sharing insights on past performance.

"A culture of data-sharing means a more successful enterprise."

—Chris Atkins, Director, Indiana Office of Management and Budget

By augmenting existing research efforts, analytics has the potential to uncover new approaches to stubborn problems. "People have been trying to improve performance and outcomes related to the public sector, and in particular, in areas like human services," continues Brandt. They do research, take the best of it and use it to model policy changes. "Analytics gives us the opportunity to show that data is a powerful component to be used," he says, "to make decisions and to improve outcomes."

Atkins says the state is now developing additional predictive analytics projects related to achieving the goals that Gov. Pence set out in his roadmap.

Transforming Service Delivery

Three other projects in the state's data analytics program aim to improve transparency, so that policymakers and the public alike are able to more easily see government performance. Indiana is using the in-memory platform and data visualization tools to make data more visible. For one project, the OMB is working with agency leaders to collect data for specific KPIs tied to each state agency's performance. Another involves developing an executive dashboard system that will enable state leaders to scan these metrics and know when they change.

A related project includes the launch, in July 2014, of an online Management and Performance Hub (MPH) to share performance data in sectors tied to Gov. Pence's roadmap, including private sector employment, elementary students' reading skills and the percentage of children who are at risk of going hungry. The measures are posted on the MPH Web site, with graphs and charts that set baselines for comparison as data is added or updated.

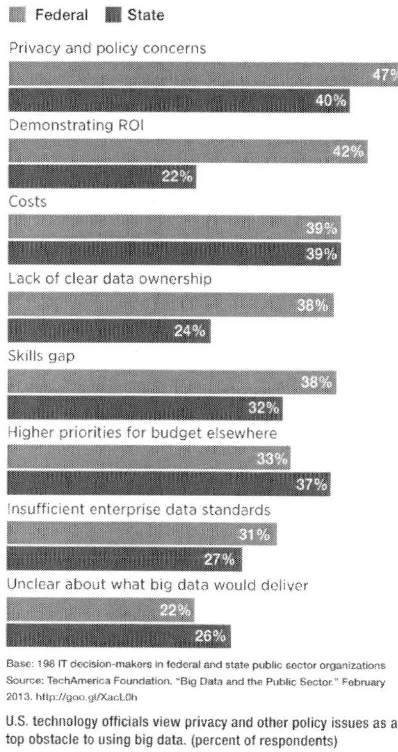

Figure 5. Breaking down Barriers.

Taken as a whole, these moves have attracted the attention of government innovation watchers like Stephen Goldsmith, a former Indianapolis mayor who is a professor at Harvard's Kennedy School of Government. Goldsmith writes: "With the launch of MPH and strong central leadership, Indiana stands to become a model for other governments looking to embed data throughout their operations and tap the power of data analytics to save money and transform service delivery."[30]

---

[30] Goldsmith, Stephen. "How Indiana Is Supercharging Data for Efficiency." Governing, June 18, 2014. http://goo.gl/kC4pnY.

About Forbes Insights

Forbes Insights is the strategic research and thought leadership practice of Forbes Media, publisher of Forbes magazine and Forbes.com, whose combined media properties reach nearly 50 million business decision-makers worldwide on a monthly basis.

Bruce Rogers
Chief Insights Officer

Brian McLeod
Director, North America

Writer: Michael S. Goldberg is an independent business and technology writer and editor based in the Boston area.

REAL-TIME ORGANIZATIONS MAKE DECISIONS IN THE MOMENT

Forbes Insights interviewed Steve Lucas, President, Platform Solutions, SAP SE, about transforming operations with real-time insights.

What Does It Mean to Be a Real-Time Organization?

Being a real-time organization means being aware of the key factors that will impact your decisions and being able to make a decision in the moment that matters. In most public sector agencies today, decision-makers have to wait for batch processes to run. When batch technology is replaced with real-time processing, however, organizations can obtain in-the-moment policy insights instantaneously. They can use those insights to improve performance, deliver services to constituents more efficiently and develop innovative approaches to policy goals. That is why the SAP HANA platform exists: to enable organizations do business in the moment.

> "We're unlocking the true potential for innovation through new business processes and models: real-time innovation."
>
> —Steve Lucas, President, Platform Solutions, Sap Se

Where Do You See the Most Value for Different Organizations?

The value comes from three main drivers. First, we reduce the complexity of the systems required to produce your existing results. This was one of the key motivations in designing SAP HANA: massive IT simplification. You can use the platform to feed data from all different sources into one system. Second, we enable agility by giving customers the ability to get real-time insight for decision-making. Third, we're unlocking the true potential for innovation through new business processes and models: the real-time innovation.

As You Look Ahead, What New Ways of Serving Constituents Do You Envision?

Our SAP HANA platform not only can enable customers to make decisions for today, but it also provides a powerful predictive engine. Most organizations make decisions by looking in the rearview mirror. But the rearview mirror is tiny compared to the windshield looking forward. Organizations will start to build forward-looking decisions into their operating models.

What Is Your Best Advice to Organizations That Want to Start Their Real-Time Transformation?

It is not just about the technology. SAP HANA is extraordinarily innovative, but the first thing we do is look at where the opportunities are to transform business processes. Then we spend time with customers rethinking how those processes are designed, and how to remodel them. You have to start at zero: What would you do if you didn't have to wait for information? If you don't have to wait, there's an opportunity for massive reinvention and value creation across industries.

To learn more about using SAP Analytics, visit www.sap.com/analytics

To learn more about SAP's Public Sector offerings, visit www.sap.com/solution/industry/public-sector.html

Johnson & Johnson
SERVICES, INC.

Jane M. Adams
Vice President
U.S. Federal Government Affairs

1350 Eye Street, N.W.
Suite 1210
Washington, DC 20005-3305
Telephone: (202) 589-1000

September 27, 2018

The Honorable Greg Walden
2125 Rayburn House Office Building
Washington, DC 20515

Dear Chairman Walden,

I am writing to you on behalf of Johnson & Johnson in support of the *Preventing Maternal Deaths Act* and to thank the Energy and Commerce Health Subcommittee for holding the hearing, "Better Data and Better Outcomes: Reducing Maternal Mortality in the U.S.," to call attention to this complex and wide-ranging problem. We believe this hearing is a positive step forward to help address a worsening health crisis affecting families across the country.

In just 14 years (2000 to 2014), America has suffered a staggering 26 percent increase in its maternal mortality rate, many of which occur from mostly preventable causes like preeclampsia and obstetric hemorrhage. Of nations with advanced economies, the United States stands alone in experiencing increases in mortality rates. Other countries also seeing increases are South Sudan and the Democratic Republic of the Congo.

Along with the American College of Obstetricians and Gynecologists, the American College of Nurse-Midwives, and the March of Dimes, Johnson & Johnson believes that a crucial part of the U.S. solution to this problem includes utilizing higher quality data, and expert review of maternal death cases by effective maternal mortality review committees (MMRCs). MMRCs study local maternal death cases with the goal of identifying ways to make pregnancies safer, prevent loss of life, and ultimately save families from this tragedy.

Congress can advance the health of mothers and families by working for swift passage of the Preventing Maternal Deaths Act, which will commit $58 million through the Public Health Service Act to support states and to establish and improve maternal mortality review committees helping to prevent pregnancy related deaths and reduce disparities in care.

We are pleased to support this legislation, because Johnson & Johnson is committed to changing the trajectory of health for humanity and believe good health is the foundation of vibrant lives, thriving communities and forward progress. That's why for more than 130 years, Johnson & Johnson has aimed to keep people well at every age and every stage of life. Today, as the world's largest and most broadly-based health care company, we are committed to using our reach and size for good. Working together, we can work to reduce the number of maternal mortality deaths in the U.S. Please don't hesitate to reach out to me for further information.

Sincerely,

Jane M. Adams

Jane M. Adams
Vice President, U.S. Federal Affairs

In: Maternal Mortality
Editor: Mathias T. Gregersen
ISBN: 978-1-53618-161-6

Chapter 3

THE IMPACT OF THE PREGNANCY CHECKBOX AND MISCLASSIFICATION ON MATERNAL MORTALITY TRENDS IN THE UNITED STATES, 1999–2017*

Lauren M. Rossen, Lindsay S. Womack, Donna L. Hoyert, Robert N. Anderson and Sayeedha F.G. Uddin

National Center for Health Statistics
Jennifer H. Madans, PhD, Acting Director
Amy M. Branum, PhD, Acting Associate Director for Science

Division of Research and Methodology
Jennifer D. Parker, PhD, Director
Donald Malec, PhD, Associate Director for Science

---

* This is an edited, reformatted and augmented version of U.S. Department of Health and Human Services; Centers for Disease Control and Prevention; National Center for Health Statistics, Publication No. 2020–1428; Series 3, Number 44, dated January 2020.

Division of Vital Statistics
Steven Schwartz, PhD, Director
Hanyu Ni, PhD, MPH, Associate Director for Science

Abstract

Background

National maternal mortality rates (MMRs) using mortality data from the National Vital Statistics System have not been reported since 2007 due to the staggered implementation of the 2003 U.S. Standard Certificate of Death between 2003 and 2017, which added a checkbox to determine pregnancy status at the time of death. This chapter evaluates the impact of the staggered implementation of the pregnancy checkbox and potential outcome misclassification on MMRs and related trends from 1999 through 2017.

Methods

Log-binomial regression models were used to examine the impact of the staggered implementation of the pregnancy checkbox by states over time and to predict MMRs under two alternative scenarios: (1) assuming that no states had the checkbox at any point, and (2) assuming that all states had the checkbox from 1999 through 2017. The impact of the checkbox and related trends over time were examined by age, race and Hispanic origin, state of occurrence, and causes of maternal death. Sensitivity analyses examined the impact of outcome misclassification.

Results

The implementation of the checkbox was associated with an increased identification of maternal deaths. Averaging over the period 2003–2017, the checkbox resulted in an MMR increase of 9.6 deaths per 100,000 live births (95% confidence interval: 8.6–10.6). The average impact of the checkbox adoption was greater for women aged 40 and over, non-Hispanic black women, and for certain causes of death.

Accounting for the checkbox, predicted MMRs did not change significantly from 1999 through 2017, although trends varied by subgroup (age, race and Hispanic origin, cause of death).

Conclusion

Estimated trends suggest that the observed increases in MMRs from 1999 through 2017 reported in the literature were largely due to the staggered implementation of the checkbox. Potential misclassification of pregnancy status using the pregnancy checkbox likely also contributed, which disproportionately inflated MMRs among women aged 40 and over.

Keywords: death certificate, epidemiologic methods, maternal death, National Vital Statistics System

INTRODUCTION

Maternal mortality is a critical indicator of population health in both the United States and internationally [1–3]. Monitoring maternal mortality over time is important to evaluate progress in improving maternal health in the United States, to make international comparisons, and to examine differences and inequities by demographic subgroup [3]. Substantial disparities in maternal mortality exist by race and Hispanic origin and age in the United States [4–6]. Maternal and pregnancy-related mortality rates for non-Hispanic black women are approximately three times the rates for non-Hispanic white women, while women aged 40 and over have the highest maternal mortality rates compared with other age groups [4, 6, 7].

The National Vital Statistics System (NVSS) is the official source for U.S. maternal mortality statistics used in international, state, and demographic comparisons. NVSS is used to tabulate the number of maternal deaths, defined by the World Health Organization (WHO) as the "death of a woman while pregnant or within 42 days of termination of pregnancy, irrespective of the duration and site of the pregnancy, from any cause related to or aggravated by the pregnancy or its management but not from accidental or incidental causes" [3]. Of note, this is different from the Centers for Disease Control and Prevention definition of pregnancy-related deaths, defined as the death of a woman while pregnant or within 1 year of pregnancy termination— regardless of the duration or site of the pregnancy—from any cause related to or aggravated by the pregnancy or its management, but not from accidental or incidental causes; and from pregnancy-associated deaths, defined as all deaths during pregnancy or within 1 year of pregnancy, regardless of cause.

Examinations of maternal deaths prior to 2000 suggested substantial underreporting of maternal deaths in NVSS [8–12]. To improve identification of maternal deaths, a pregnancy question was added to the 2003 revision of the U.S. Standard Certificate of Death. This pregnancy question includes a series of checkboxes to determine whether female decedents were currently or recently pregnant (within 42 days, or 43 days to 1 year). Jurisdictions adopted this revision at different times between 2003 and 2017, making it difficult to estimate national-level trends in maternal mortality over this time period [13, 14]. Subsequently, national maternal mortality rates (MMRs) have not been reported since 2007. Studies have suggested that the pregnancy checkbox resulted in the identification of more maternal or pregnancy-associated deaths [8, 15]. A companion report examines the impact of the pregnancy checkbox by recoding cause of death without consideration of the checkbox, using data on maternal deaths from 2015 through 2016 [15]. Findings suggest that the number of maternal deaths was approximately three times higher when using information from the checkbox compared with the recoded data without considering the checkbox [15]. Differences were seen in the magnitude of the impact of the checkbox by maternal age, race and Hispanic origin, and cause of death. Specifically, among women aged 40 and over, the number of maternal deaths reported with the checkbox was more than 14 times higher than the number reported without using information from the checkbox. That companion report offers additional detail about the coding of maternal deaths and differences in the impact of the checkbox by cause of death.

Given the substantial impact of the checkbox on the identification of maternal deaths, estimating trends in maternal mortality considering its staggered implementation across the United States has proved challenging. Several studies have attempted to account for the checkbox in examinations of recent trends in maternal mortality. MacDorman et al. examined trends from 2000 through 2014 and reported that MMRs (maternal deaths per 100,000 live births) increased by nearly 30%, from 18.8 in 2000 to 23.8 in 2014; however, these estimates excluded California and Texas, and correction factors (to account for changes in measurement associated with the checkbox) were calculated based on 24 states and the District of Columbia [14]. Joseph et al. suggested that most of the increase in MMRs from 1993 through 2014 was due to the implementation of the checkbox and that increases were limited to nonspecific causes of maternal death [16]. Davis et al. reported that 90% of the increase from 1998–2002 through 2008–2012 was due to the implementation of the pregnancy checkbox, comparing a subset of 23 states that adopted the checkbox with a group of 11 states that had not [17]. Another study suggested that only 31% of the increase in MMRs from 1997 through 2012 was attributable to the 2003 death certificate revision [18] but was limited to the 36 states that had adopted the revision by 2012. Because prior studies examining the impact of the pregnancy checkbox have typically looked at subsets of states [4, 14, 17], the impact of the checkbox on national trends since 1999 remains unclear; 2017 is the first year that all states have adopted the 2003 revision of the certificate, allowing for examination of national-level data.

Although pregnancy checkboxes have been found to identify a greater percentage of deaths during or following pregnancy [8, 19], some reports suggest that approximately 14% of pregnancy-associated deaths had no verifiable evidence of pregnancy [20]. Therefore, misclassification of pregnancy status on death certificates may have contributed to biased trend estimates [19, 21, 22]. An examination of Texas MMRs reported increases from 2006 through 2015, but the extent to which the increase was driven by overreporting of maternal deaths was unclear, particularly among women aged 40 and over [23]. A review of 147 maternal deaths in Texas suggested that approximately one-half of obstetric-coded deaths had no evidence of pregnancy within 42 days of death, with 67% of the deaths among women aged 35 and over showing no evidence of pregnancy [24]. Davis et al. also suggested that a high degree of misclassification of pregnancy status among women aged 40 and over may explain the increasing trends seen among this age group. The impact of potential misclassification of pregnancy status on MMRs among all states incorporating the pregnancy checkbox has not been explored.

The objectives of this analysis were to (1) quantify the impact of the staggered implementation of the pregnancy checkbox on MMRs overall and by maternal age, race and Hispanic origin, cause of death, and state; (2) estimate trends in MMRs from 1999 through 2017, accounting for the checkbox, overall and by maternal age, race and Hispanic origin, and cause of death; and (3) examine the impact of potential misclassification of pregnancy status on the death certificate on trends in MMRs from 1999 through 2017.

Methods

Data

Data on maternal deaths and births were drawn from NVSS for the years 1999 through 2017. Maternal deaths for each year were identified using International Classification of Diseases, 10th Revision (ICD–10) underlying-cause codes A34, O00–O95, and O98–O99, consistent with the WHO definition. Late maternal deaths (those occurring more than 42 days following pregnancy) were identified using the underlying-cause codes O96 and O97, and analyzed separately. Denominators for maternal mortality rates were calculated from NVSS birth data for 1999 through 2017 [25]. Maternal deaths and corresponding numbers of live births were aggregated by year, state of occurrence, race and Hispanic origin (non-Hispanic white, non-Hispanic black, Hispanic, non-Hispanic other), and age group (under 15, 15–19, 20–24, 25–29, 30–34, 35–39, 40 and over). State of occurrence, rather than residence, was used because the death certificate information (and consequently, the pregnancy checkbox) is collected using the certificate issued by state of occurrence.

Causes of Maternal Death

Prior studies suggested that the impact of the pregnancy checkbox varied by cause of death [4, 16]. Subsequently, analyses examined the impact of the checkbox and related trends over time by various causes (and groups of causes) of maternal deaths:

- O00–O07: Pregnancy with abortive outcomes
- O10–O16: Edema, proteinuria and hypertensive disorders in pregnancy, childbirth and the puerperium
- O20–O29: Other maternal disorders predominantly related to pregnancy
- O26.6: Liver disorders in pregnancy, childbirth and the puerperium
- O26.8: Other specified pregnancy-related conditions
- O30–O48: Maternal care related to the fetus and amniotic cavity and possible delivery problems
- O60–O75: Complications of labor and delivery
- O85–O92: Complications predominantly related to the puerperium
- O95–O99: Other obstetric conditions not elsewhere classified (including late maternal deaths)
- O95, O98–O99: Other obstetric conditions not elsewhere classified (excluding late maternal deaths)
- O96–O97: Late maternal deaths
- O99.3: Mental disorders and diseases of the nervous system complicating pregnancy, childbirth and the puerperium
- O99.4: Diseases of the circulatory system complicating pregnancy, childbirth and the puerperium
- O99.5: Diseases of the respiratory system complicating pregnancy, childbirth and the puerperium

- O99.8: Other specified diseases and conditions complicating pregnancy, childbirth and the puerperium
- Direct causes [26]
- Indirect causes [26]
- O26.8, O95, O99.8: Nonspecific causes
- A34, O00–O92: Alternative grouping of direct causes [4]
- O98–O99: Alternative grouping of indirect causes [4]
- A34, O00–O95: Alternative grouping of direct causes [15]

Statistical Analysis

Objective 1: Quantify the Impact of the Staggered Implementation of the Pregnancy Checkbox on MMRs

A regression-discontinuity approach was used to examine the impact of adopting the pregnancy checkbox on maternal mortality rates overall, by demographic group, and by cause of death. Regression-discontinuity designs can be used to examine the causal effects of a given intervention when the exposure to that intervention is based on a specific threshold [27]. Assuming that observations immediately below and above the threshold are otherwise similar, the difference at the threshold corresponds to the causal effect estimate of that intervention [27–29]. By examining MMRs immediately prior to and after the implementation of the checkbox, the impact of the checkbox on MMRs can be estimated.

First, a variable was created by subtracting the year that states revised their certificates [30] from the year of death. This variable represents time since revision year, equal to zero in the year that the state revised. This variable represents the threshold value used in a regression-discontinuity analysis—states and other factors related to maternal mortality are assumed to be otherwise similar immediately before and after the revision, the major difference being the addition of the pregnancy checkbox. To examine the impact of the checkbox visually, MMRs were plotted against the "time since revision" variable using fractional polynomial prediction plots in Stata 14 SE (College Station, Tex.), which allows for nonlinear trends. Plots were limited to show trends within plus or minus 4 years of the revision, with the discontinuity between the lines pre- and postrevision (when "time since revision" is equal to zero) representing the impact of the checkbox on MMRs. Four years before and after the implementation of the checkbox are shown to visually inspect any potential temporal trends prior to or following the checkbox.

Frequency-weighted log-binomial regression models with robust standard errors were implemented using Stata 14 SE to examine whether the impact of the checkbox differed by various demographic characteristics. These models also were used to estimate trends over time, accounting for the staggered adoption of the pregnancy checkbox by states from 2003 through 2017. MMRs were modeled as a function of revision status, state of occurrence, year, age group, and race and Hispanic origin. Additionally, interactions between revision status and state, age group, and race and Hispanic origin were included to allow for the impact of the checkbox to vary by these factors. Interactions between year and state of occurrence, age group, and race and Hispanic origin allowed temporal trends to vary by these factors. Finally, models including indicators for whether a given state had a pregnancy question prior to the checkbox implementation (Alabama, Florida, Illinois, Indiana, Iowa, Kentucky, Louisiana, Maryland, Minnesota, Mississippi, Missouri, Nebraska, New Jersey, New Mexico, New York City, New York State, North Dakota, Texas, and Virginia), and for when coding was centralized at the National Center for Health Statistics (NCHS) in 2011, also were explored to assess whether MMRs and the impact of the revision varied by these factors. California was not included in the set of states with pregnancy questions prior to the checkbox implementation, because it uses a question that is inconsistent with the 2003 standard certificate, asking about pregnancy status in the past 12 months.

Average marginal effects were used to estimate the change in the MMRs associated with the revision overall, and by age group, race and Hispanic origin, state of occurrence, cause-of-death grouping, and whether the state had a pregnancy question on the death certificate prior to the revision. All analyses were conducted using Stata 14 SE, and no adjustments were made for multiple comparisons.

Objective 2: Estimate Trends in MMRs from 1999 through 2017, Accounting for the Checkbox

To examine trends from 1999 through 2017, maternal mortality rates were predicted based on two scenarios: (1) assuming that no states had adopted the checkbox and (2) assuming that all states had implemented the checkbox throughout the entire study period. Observed and predicted trends were estimated overall and by age group, race and Hispanic origin, state of occurrence, and cause-of-death group. Average marginal effects were used to estimate the linear time trends overall and by group, adjusted for the factors included in the models (e.g., age, race and Hispanic origin, state, revision status). These average marginal effects represent the estimated annual absolute change in the MMRs under the two scenarios described previously, controlling for sociodemographic factors such as age, race and Hispanic origin, and state.

Objective 3: Examine the Impact of Potential Misclassification of Pregnancy Status on the Death Certificate on MMR Trends from 1999 through 2017

Several additional analyses were conducted to examine the potential impact of misclassification [31, 32] of pregnancy status on MMRs and related trends (see Appendix I for more details). Prior studies have suggested that the pregnancy checkbox resulted in many deaths being classified as maternal (or pregnancy-associated) when there was no evidence of pregnancy, with false-positive rates as high as 50% [13, 17–24, 33–35]. Other studies have described substantial false-negative rates (failure to identify pregnancy on death certificates) both before and after the implementation of the checkbox [8, 12, 22, 34, 36, 37].

Accounting for a Certain Percentage of Death Certificates Where a Pregnancy Checkbox May Have Been Selected in Error

To determine a plausible range for the error rate, the percentage of records where one of the pregnancy checkboxes was selected (either currently pregnant, pregnant within 42 days, or pregnant 43 days to 1 year) among women of ages where pregnancy would be implausible (age 10 years and under or 55 and over) was calculated by state of occurrence. There was variability by state in the percentage of records where this occurred, with the largest percentages in North Dakota, California, New Jersey, Oklahoma, Michigan, New York State (excluding New York City), Kentucky, Tennessee, Utah, the District of Columbia, New Hampshire, Rhode Island, and Texas (ranging from 0.05% to 0.34%; see Table I).

Models were run assuming that 0.25%, 0.50%, or 1.00% of death certificates for female decedents had a pregnancy checkbox selected in error (currently pregnant or pregnant within 42 days). These percentages were used to adjust the observed numbers of maternal deaths. For each state, age, and racial or Hispanic-origin group, these percentages (expressed as proportions) were multiplied by the total number of deaths among females aged 15–44 in that group to estimate the number of overall death records that may have a checkbox marked in error. These numbers were subtracted from the observed numbers of maternal deaths in each stratum (among states and years where the checkbox applied), and the models were refit. Because more deaths occur among older women, this adjustment had a disproportionate impact on MMRs among older age groups, even assuming a constant error rate of 0.25%, 0.50%, or 1.00%.

Adjusting for Outcome Misclassification

Additionally, MMRs were corrected for potential outcome misclassification based on prior validation studies examining the accuracy of death record data in identifying maternal deaths, conducted before the implementation of the checkbox [8, 9, 11, 12, 38] and after [13, 17–24, 33–35]. These studies have provided a range of values for the sensitivity (Se) of death certificate data (the proportion of true maternal deaths captured in death certificate data), predictive value positive (PVP; the proportion of maternal deaths determined using death certificate data that are true maternal deaths), or false-positive rates (the proportion of maternal deaths determined using death certificate data that are not maternal deaths).

A data visualization tool (available from: https://www.cdc.gov/nchs/maternal-mortality/dashboard/) was developed to explore the impact of potential misclassification on MMR trends overall and by demographic group, allowing users to vary Se and false-positive rates within plausible ranges (0.4–1.0 for Se, 0.00–0.75 for false-positive rates). The following formula was used to adjust the predicted MMRs based on Se and PVP values (where PVP is equal to 1–false- positive rate; see Appendix I for more detail):

$$\#\ \text{Maternal Deaths}_{adj} = \frac{\#\ \text{Maternal Deaths}_{obs} \bullet \text{PVP}}{\text{Se}} \quad (1)$$

Because the Se and PVP values differed before and after the implementation of the checkbox, values defined for the period prior to the checkbox implementation were applied to the predicted MMRs assuming that no states adopted the checkbox, while values defined for the period after the checkbox implementation were applied to the predicted MMRs assuming that all states had adopted the checkbox throughout 1999–2017.

Falsification Test: Nonmaternal Causes of Death

Finally, the impact of the checkbox was examined for several nonmaternal causes of death, including unintentional injuries, suicide, homicide, drug overdose, and unknown or ill-specified (R99). These are not maternal causes of death according to the WHO definition, and so, should not necessarily have changed because of the adoption of the checkbox. However, in some cases, deaths due to these causes may be coded as a maternal death due to ICD–10 coding rules relating to what information appears on the death certificate and where it appears [15, 39, 40]. To explore whether changes in these nonmaternal causes were a result of the implementation of the checkbox, two sets of models were run.

First, the percentage of overall deaths among women of reproductive age (15–44 years) due to these causes was modeled using the same frequency-weighted log-binomial models described previously. The estimated impact of the checkbox refers to the change in the percentage of deaths among women of reproductive age due to these five causes. Second, as a falsification test, these same models were run for females under age 10 or 55–59, where there should be no impact of the checkbox because it does not apply to these age groups in determining the underlying cause-of-death code. If changes in the percentages of deaths among these groups occurred due to these causes, then it would suggest that there are factors confounding the estimates of the impact of the pregnancy checkbox (e.g., the adoption of electronic death registration systems, or other data quality improvements that may have occurred at the same time as the adoption of the revised standard certificate). Finally, if there were declines in the percentages of deaths due to these external causes (and unknown or ill-specified causes) among women of reproductive age associated with the implementation of the checkbox, then it could suggest that the coding changes instituted with the implementation of the checkbox resulted in a certain percentage of these deaths being assigned a maternal cause of death.

RESULTS

The Impact of the Implementation of the Pregnancy Checkbox on MMRs

Overall, the addition of the pregnancy checkbox on the 2003 standard death certificate, which was implemented in staggered fashion across the United States from 2003 through 2017, was associated with an average increase of 9.6 maternal deaths per 100,000 live births (95% confidence interval [CI]: 8.6–10.6). Figure 1 shows the trends in MMRs prior to and immediately after the implementation of the checkbox.

The average impact of the revision varied by maternal age, race and Hispanic origin, and state of occurrence. For females aged 15–34, the implementation of the checkbox resulted in an increase in the age-specific MMRs ranging from 3.7 (95% CI: 1.7–5.7) among teenagers (ages 15–19) to 6.0 (95% CI: 3.9–8.0) among women (ages 30–34) (Table 1; Figures 2 and 3). For women aged 35–39, MMRs increased by 13.9 (95% CI: 9.7–18.0). The impact of the checkbox on MMRs among women over 40 was much larger than for other age groups, with an increase of 145.3 (95% CI: 127.6–163.1). By race and Hispanic origin, the checkbox was associated with increases of 6.2 (95% CI: 4.3–8.1) among Hispanic women, 7.1 (95% CI: 4.2–10.0) among non-Hispanic women of other races, 8.6 (95% CI: 7.5–9.7) among non-Hispanic white women, and 19.6 (95% CI: 15.3–24.0) among non-Hispanic black women (Table 1; Figure 4).

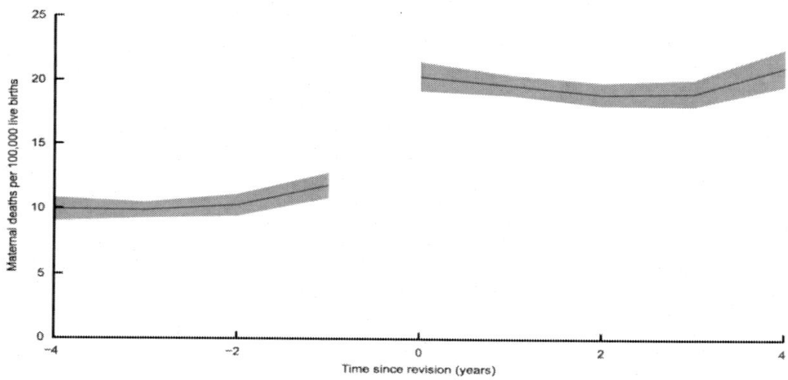

Note: Figure was generated using Fractional polynomial prediction plots in Stata 14 SE, with shaded areas corresponding to 95% confidence intervals.
Source: NCHS, National Vital Statistics System.

Figure 1. Average change in maternal mortality rates associated with the pregnancy checkbox implementation: United States, 2003–2017.

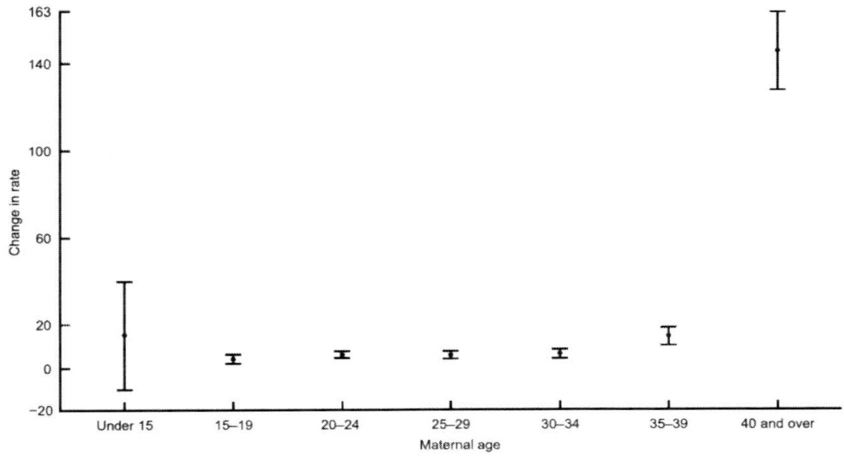

Source: NCHS, National Vital Statistics System.

Figure 2. Average change in maternal mortality rates associated with the pregnancy checkbox implementation, by age: United States, 2003–2017.

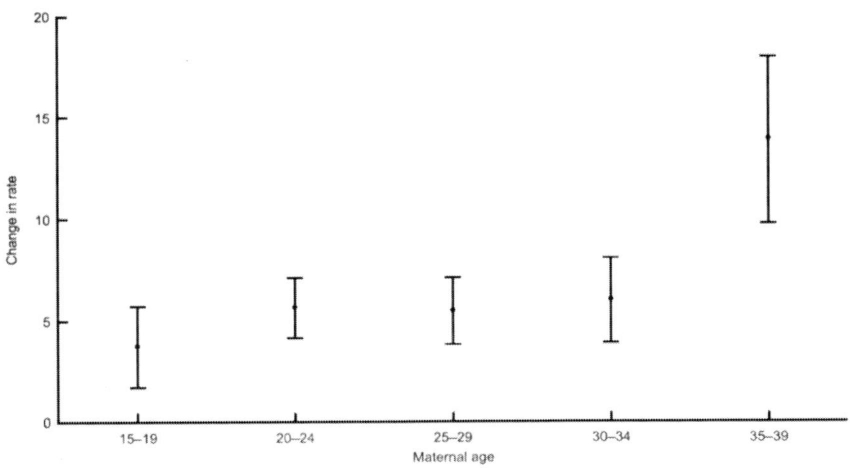

Source: NCHS, National Vital Statistics System.

Figure 3. Average change in maternal mortality rates associated with the pregnancy checkbox implementation among females aged 15–39, by age: United States, 2003–2017.

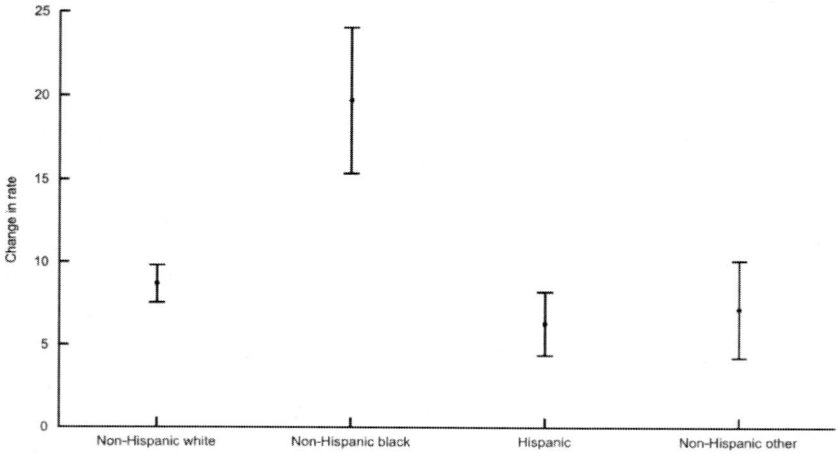

Source: NCHS, National Vital Statistics System.

Figure 4. Average change in maternal mortality rates associated with the pregnancy checkbox implementation, by race and Hispanic origin: United States, 2003–2017.

The impact of the checkbox was smaller among states that had a question about pregnancy status prior to the adoption of the revised standard certificate (8.1, 95% CI: 6.8–9.4) than among states that did not have a pregnancy question (9.8, 95% CI: 8.7–10.9). Additionally, the impact of the revision was larger after the coding of cause of death was centralized at NCHS in 2011 (10.9, 95% CI: 9.5–12.2) compared with before (9.0, 95% CI: 8.0–10.0).

Differences by state of occurrence were seen in the impact of the checkbox, with most states exhibiting increases in MMRs, except Maryland, where the MMR declined (Figure 5; Table II). The point estimates for Mississippi, Hawaii, Wisconsin, Nebraska, Pennsylvania, Nevada, and Rhode Island also indicated that MMRs declined as a result of the checkbox, but the CIs around these estimated changes were wide, and the 95% CI bounds were compatible with the possibility that MMRs increased or did not change as a result of the checkbox.

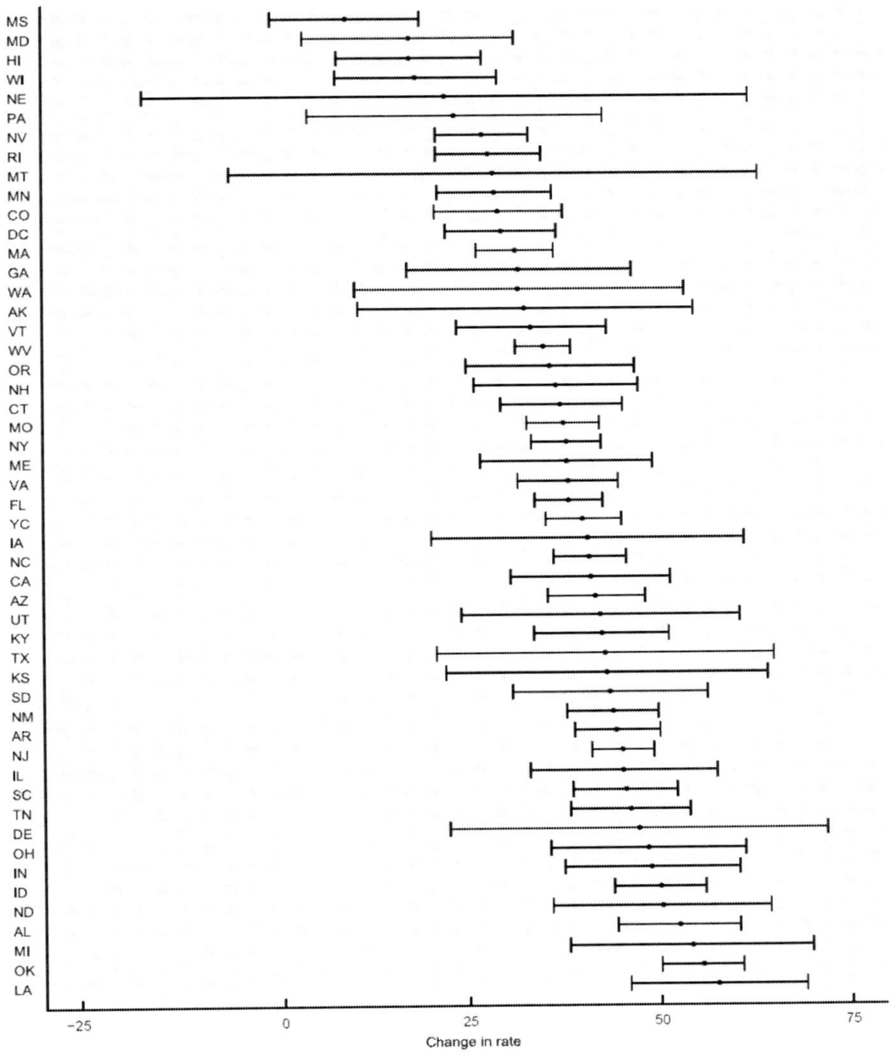

Note: Wyoming was excluded as the estimate was highly unstable (95% confidence interval: -22.48-191.33).

Source: NCHS, National Vital Statistics System.

Figure 5. Average change in maternal mortality rates associated with the pregnancy checkbox implementation, by state of occurrence: United States, 2003–2017.

The largest increases in MMRs as a result of the checkbox were seen in Louisiana, Oklahoma, Michigan, Alabama, Idaho, Indiana, Ohio, Tennessee, South Carolina, Illinois, New Jersey, and Arkansas (all increased by more than 15 maternal deaths per 100,000 live births). Wyoming, North Dakota, and Delaware also exhibited increases of 15 or more, but the CIs around these estimates were wide due to the small number of events in these states, and the 95% CI bounds were compatible with the possibility that MMRs either declined or did not change as a result of the checkbox.

Observed and Predicted MMR Trends from 1999 through 2017, Accounting for the Checkbox

Figure 6 illustrates the overall trends in the observed MMRs and in the predicted MMRs, assuming that no states had adopted the checkbox during this time period, and in the predicted MMRs, assuming that all states had adopted the checkbox during this time period. Both with and without the checkbox, no significant change in the MMRs was observed in adjusted models (−0.03, 95% CI: −0.09–0.03, $p = 0.307$; 0.04, 95% CI: −0.07–0.15, $p = 0.459$, respectively). Without the checkbox, estimated MMRs were 10.3 maternal deaths per 100,000 live births in 1999 and 12.8 in 2017 (Table IV). Assuming that all states had adopted the checkbox in 1999, estimated MMRs were 21.2 in 1999 and 23.5 in 2017. Of note, unadjusted trend estimates accounting only for revision status by state showed an average annual increase in MMRs both without the checkbox (0.12, 95% CI: 0.06–0.18, $p < 0.001$) and with the checkbox (0.22, 95% CI: 0.12–0.32, $p < 0.001$).

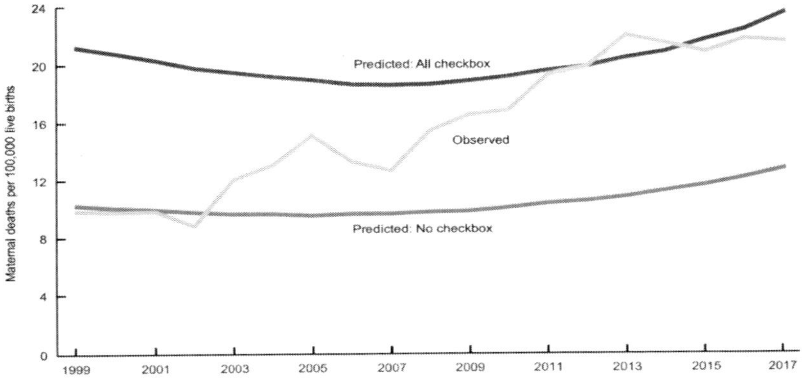

Note: Models were adjusted for age group, race and Hispanic origin, and state of occurrence, and included interactions between these factors and year as well as revision status.

Source: NCHS, National Vital Statistics System.

Figure 6. Observed and predicted maternal mortality rates: United States, 1999–2017.

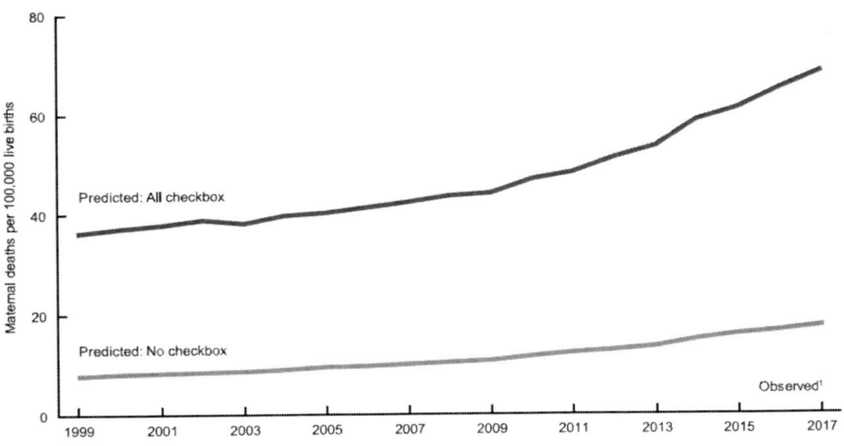

[1]Observed rates suppressed when the number of deaths is fewer than 20 (all years).

Note: Models were adjusted for age group, race and Hispanic origin, and state of occurrence, and included interactions between these factors and year as well as revision status.

Source: NCHS, National Vital Statistics System.

Figure 7. Observed and predicted maternal mortality rates among females under age 15: United States, 1999–2017.

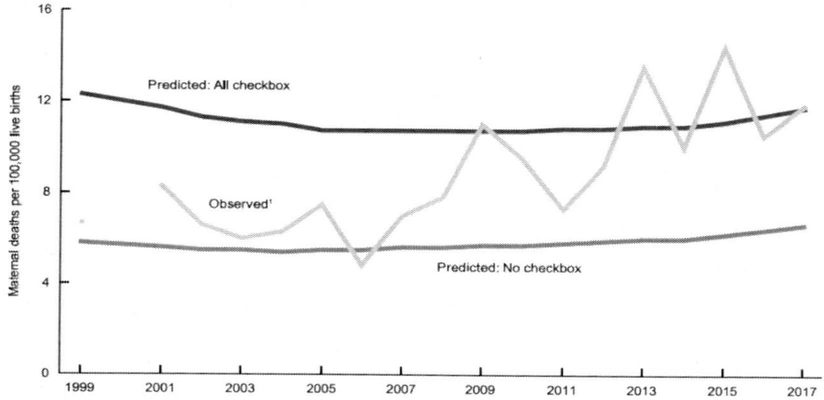

¹Observed rates suppressed when the number of deaths is fewer than 20 (in 2000).

Note: Models were adjusted for age group, race and Hispanic origin, and state of occurrence, and included interactions between these factors and year as well as revision status.

Source: NCHS, National Vital Statistics System.

Figure 8. Observed and predicted maternal mortality rates among females aged 15–19: United States, 1999–2017.

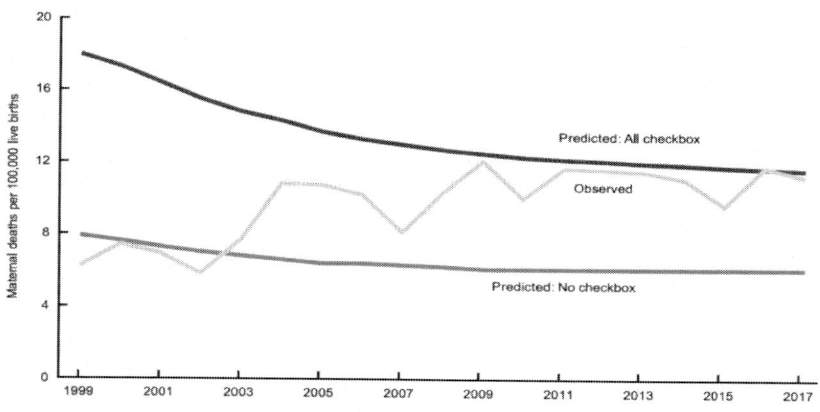

Note: Models were adjusted for age group, race and Hispanic origin, and state of occurrence, and included interactions between these factors and year as well as revision status.

Source: NCHS, National Vital Statistics System.

Figure 9. Observed and predicted maternal mortality rates among women aged 20–24: United States, 1999–2017.

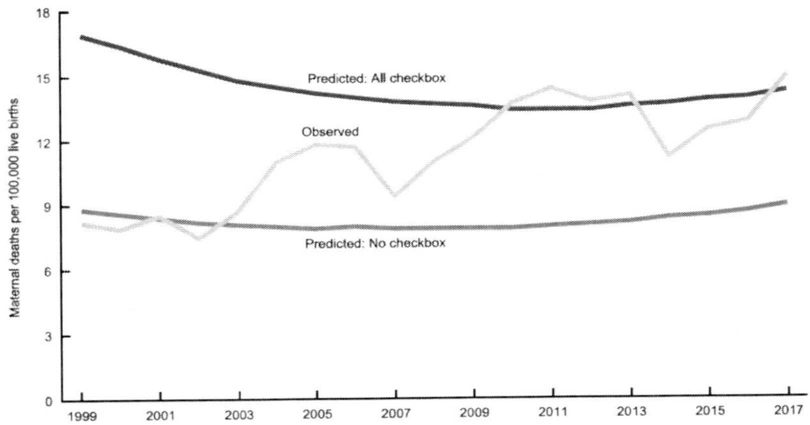

Note: Models were adjusted for age group, race and Hispanic origin, and state of occurrence, and included interactions between these factors and year as well as revision status.

Source: NCHS, National Vital Statistics System.

Figure 10. Observed and predicted maternal mortality rates among women aged 25–29: United States, 1999–2017.

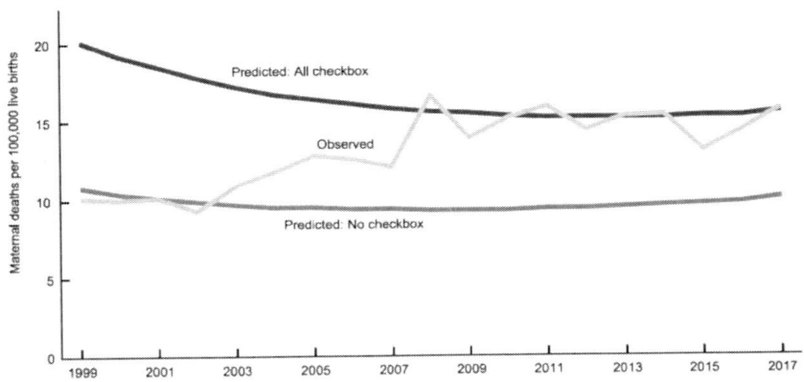

Note: Models were adjusted for age group, race and Hispanic origin, and state of occurrence, and included interactions between these factors and year as well as revision status.

Source: NCHS, National Vital Statistics System.

Figure 11. Observed and predicted maternal mortality rates among women aged 30–34: United States, 1999–2017.

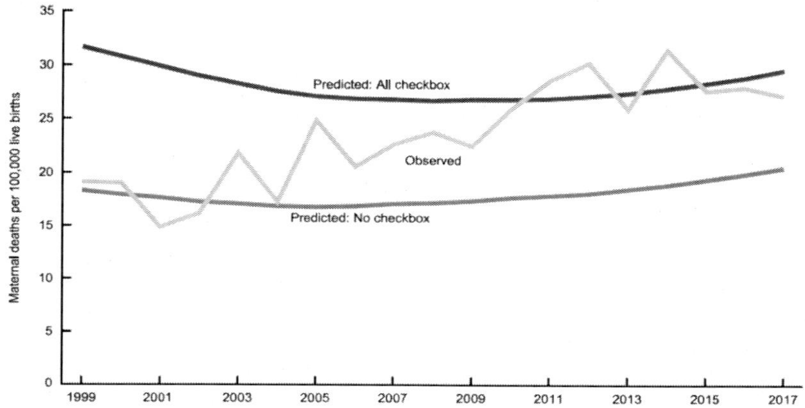

Note: Models were adjusted for age group, race and Hispanic origin, and state of occurrence, and included interactions between these factors and year as well as revision status.

Source: NCHS, National Vital Statistics System.

Figure 12. Observed and predicted maternal mortality rates among women aged 35–39: United States, 1999–2017.

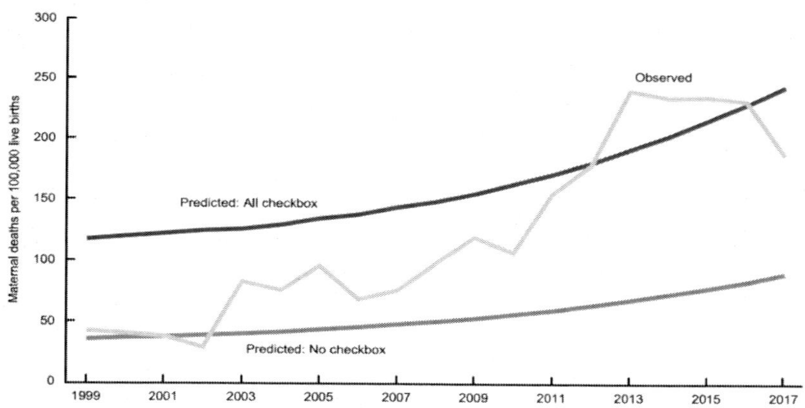

Note: Models were adjusted for age group, race and Hispanic origin, and state of occurrence, and included interactions between these factors and year as well as revision status.

Source: NCHS, National Vital Statistics System.

Figure 13. Observed and predicted maternal mortality rates among women aged 40 and over: United States, 1999–2017.

Figures 7–13 show trends by age group. No significant changes in predicted MMRs were seen with or without the checkbox for the youngest groups (under 15 and 15–19) (Table 2; Figures 7 and 8). Without the checkbox, predicted MMRs declined for women aged 20–24 (−0.1 per year, 95% CI: −0.2 – −0.0, $p = 0.001$; see Figure 9) and 30–34 (−0.2 per year, 95% CI: −0.3 – −0.1, $p = 0.002$; see Figure 11). Predicted MMRs did not change significantly for women aged 25–29 (−0.1 per year, 95% CI: −0.2–0.0, $p = 0.057$; see Figure 10) or 35–39 (−0.1 per year, 95% CI: −0.3–0.1, $p = 0.425$; see Figure 12) and increased for women aged 40 and over (2.5, 95% CI: 1.8–3.3, $p < 0.001$; see Figure 13). Assuming that all states had adopted the checkbox, trends were similar, declining for women aged 20–24 (−0.2 per year, 95% CI: −0.4 – −0.1, $p = 0.008$) and 30–34 (−0.3 per year, 95% CI: −0.5 – −0.1, $p = 0.013$). Predicted MMRs assuming that all states had adopted the checkbox did not change significantly for women aged 25–29 (−0.1 per year, 95% CI: −0.3–0.0, $p = 0.116$) and 35–39 (−0.1 per year, 95% CI: −0.5–0.3, $p = 0.552$) but increased for women aged 40 and over (7.7, 95% CI: 6.1–9.4, $p < 0.001$).

By race and Hispanic origin, predicted MMRs increased for non-Hispanic white women by 0.1 per year from 1999 through 2017 (95% CI: 0.1–0.2, $p < 0.001$) assuming no checkbox, and by 0.3 per year (95% CI: 0.2–0.5, $p < 0.001$) assuming all states had adopted the checkbox (Table 2; Figure 14). Trends declined for non-Hispanic black women, assuming that no states had adopted the checkbox (−0.3, 95% CI: −0.6 – −0.1, $p = 0.004$). Assuming that all states had adopted the checkbox, predicted MMRs among non- Hispanic black women declined by −0.4 per year (95% CI: −0.9–0.0), but this trend was not statistically significant ($p = 0.072$).

Among Hispanic women, predicted MMRs declined over time, both assuming no checkbox (–0.3, 95% CI: –0.3 – –0.2, $p < 0.001$) and assuming that all states had adopted the checkbox (–0.4, 95% CI: –0.6 – –0.2, $p < 0.001$). Trends among non-Hispanic women of other races did not change significantly with the checkbox (–0.2, 95% CI: –0.4–0.1, $p = 0.280$) or without (–0.1, 95% CI: –0.3–0.0, $p = 0.104$).

Causes of Maternal Death

The impact of the checkbox varied by maternal cause of death (Table 3). Cause-specific MMRs increased by less than 0.5 deaths per 100,000 live births because of the checkbox for the following causes (or groups of causes): pregnancy with abortive outcomes (O00–O07); edema, proteinuria and hypertensive disorders in pregnancy, childbirth and the puerperium (O10–O16); liver disorders in pregnancy, childbirth and the puerperium (O26.6); maternal care related to the fetus and amniotic cavity and possible delivery problems (O30–O48); complications of labor and delivery (O60–O75); complications predominantly related to the puerperium (O85–O92); mental disorders and diseases of the nervous system complicating pregnancy, childbirth and the puerperium (O99.3); and diseases of the respiratory system complicating pregnancy, childbirth and the puerperium (O99.5).

The impact of the checkbox was largest for indirect or nonspecific causes of death. Maternal deaths due to other obstetric conditions not elsewhere classified (O95–O99) increased by 8.3 (95% CI: 7.6–9.0) as a result of the checkbox, and nonspecific causes (O26.8, O95, O99.8) increased by 5.6 (95% CI: 5.1–6.1). While MMRs for direct causes [26] increased by 5.2 (95% CI: 4.4–6.1) as a result of the checkbox, the impact was driven by the inclusion of a nonspecific cause of death in this category, other specified pregnancy-related conditions (O26.8). Late maternal MMRs increased by 3.5 (95% CI: 3.1–3.9) as a result of the checkbox.

Trends in predicted MMRs both with and without the checkbox varied by cause of death (Table 4; Figures I–XXIII). Predicted MMRs declined significantly from 1999 through 2017 under both scenarios for the following causes of maternal death: direct causes [26] (excluding O26.8, other specified pregnancy-related conditions); pregnancy with abortive outcomes (O00–O07); edema, proteinuria and hypertensive disorders in pregnancy, childbirth and the puerperium (O10–O16); complications of labor and delivery (O60–O75); and complications predominantly related to the puerperium (O85–O92). Predicted MMRs increased under both scenarios for the following causes: other maternal disorders predominantly related to pregnancy (O20–O29), which was driven by the inclusion of other specified pregnancy-related conditions (O26.8) in this group; indirect causes [26]; late maternal deaths (O96–O97); and the group of nonspecific causes (O26.8, O95, O99.8).

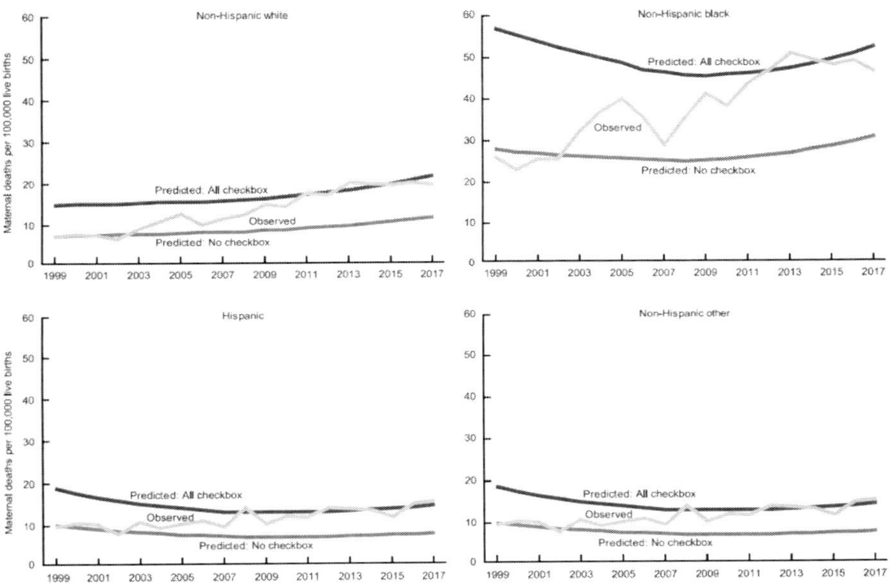

Note: Models were adjusted for age group, race and Hispanic origin, and state of occurrence, and included interactions between these factors and year as well as revision status.

Source: NCHS, National Vital Statistics System.

Figure 14. Observed and predicted maternal mortality rates, by race and Hispanic origin: United States, 1999–2017.

The Impact of Potential Misclassification of Pregnancy Status on the Death Certificate on MMR Trends from 1999 through 2017

Accounting for a Certain Percentage of Death Certificates Where a Pregnancy Checkbox May Have Been Selected in Error

Several sensitivity analyses were conducted to examine trends in MMRs over time by subgroup and cause of death, and to explore the impact of potential misclassification. Analyses accounting for varied percentages of false positives (0.25%, 0.50%, 1.00%), resulted in lower predicted MMRs from 1999 through 2017 (assuming that all states adopted the checkbox in 1999; see Figures 15-17).

The impact of the adjustment for this false-positive rate was larger for older age groups and non-Hispanic black and white women (Figures 24-30).

Adjusting for Outcome Misclassification

Results of analyses examining the impact of misclassification can be found in Table V and in the data visualization tool (available from: https://www.cdc.gov/nchs/maternal- mortality/dashboard/). For example, assuming that the values for Se before and after the implementation of the checkbox were 0.60 and 0.80, respectively, and the proportion of records that were false positives was 0.10 and 0.35, respectively, before and after the checkbox, the estimated MMRs in 2017 converged to 19.1–19.2 maternal deaths per 100,000 live births (the observed MMR was 21.6). These values for Se and proportion of false positives are within the range of previously published estimates [8, 9, 11, 13, 17–24, 33–35, 38].

Examining the predicted MMRs for women aged 40 and over and using the same values described previously, except increasing the proportion of false positives after the checkbox implementation to 0.6 (consistent with the greater degree of misclassification among this age group [17]), the predicted MMRs in 2017 were 133.9 assuming that no states had adopted the checkbox and 121.4 assuming that all states had adopted the checkbox (compared with an observed MMR of 186.1 deaths per 100,000 live births).

Falsification Test: Nonmaternal Causes Death

Finally, as a falsification test, models were run examining the impact of the pregnancy checkbox on several nonmaternal causes of death both among female decedents of reproductive age [15–44] and female decedents to whom the pregnancy checkbox does not apply (under age 10 and 55–59).

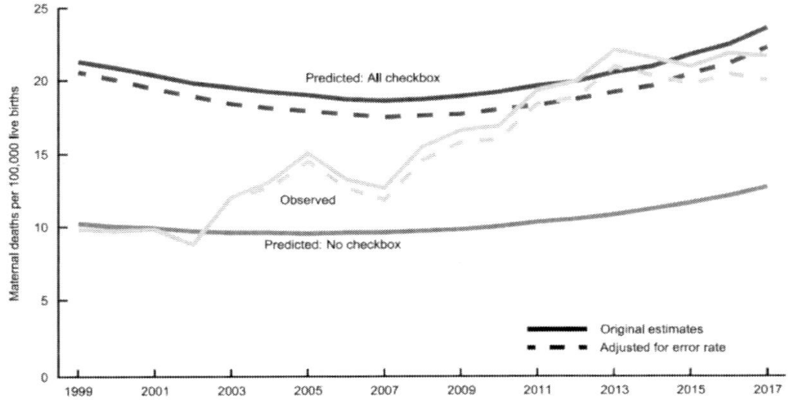

Notes: Dotted lines represent maternal mortality rates (MMRs) adjusted for fixed error rates, while solid lines depict the original predicted and observed MMRs. Models were adjusted for age group, race and Hispanic origin, and state of occurrence, and included interactions between these factors and year as well as revision status.
Source: NCHS, National Vital Statistics System.

Figure 15. Observed and predicted maternal mortality rates, adjusted for an error rate of 0.25% in the pregnancy checkbox: United States, 1999–2017.

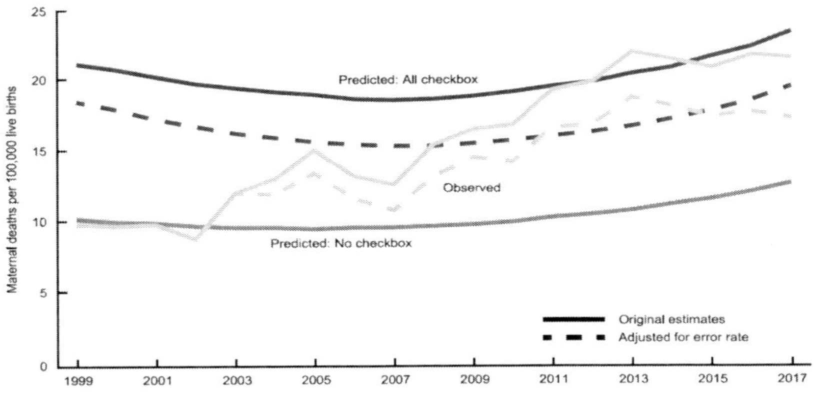

Notes: Dotted lines represent maternal mortality rates (MMRs) adjusted for fixed error rates, while solid lines depict the original predicted and observed MMRs. Models were adjusted for age group, race and Hispanic origin, and state of occurrence, and included interactions between these factors and year as well as revision status.
Source: NCHS, National Vital Statistics System.

Figure 16. Observed and predicted maternal mortality rates, adjusted for an error rate of 0.50% in the pregnancy checkbox: United States, 1999–2017.

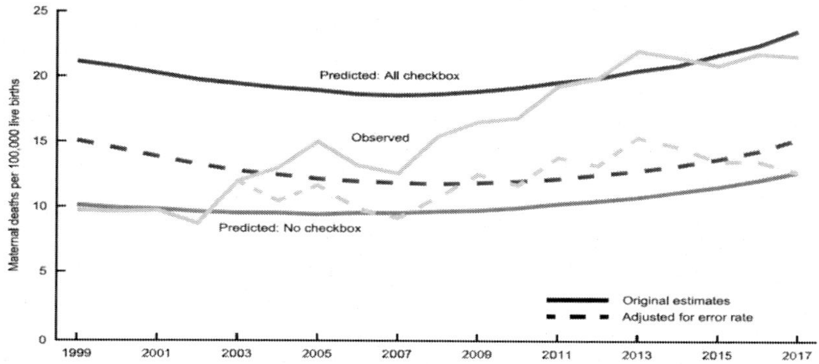

Notes: Dotted lines represent maternal mortality rates (MMRs) adjusted for fixed error rates, while solid lines depict the original predicted and observed MMRs. Models were adjusted for age group, race and Hispanic origin, and state of occurrence, and included interactions between these factors and year as well as revision status.

Source: NCHS, National Vital Statistics System.

Figure 17. Observed and predicted maternal mortality rates, adjusted for an error rate of 1.00% in the pregnancy checkbox: United States, 1999–2017.

The percentage of deaths among female decedents aged 15–44 that were due to unintentional injury, suicide, drug overdose, homicide, or unknown or ill-specified causes declined with the implementation of the pregnancy checkbox by 0.53% (95% CI: –0.85 – –0.20, $p = 0.001$) (Table 5). In contrast, there was an increase in the percentage of deaths due to these same causes among female decedents under age 10 or 55–59 (0.21, 95% CI: 0.03–0.39, $p = 0.02$). These results suggest that a small percentage of deaths due to nonmaternal causes, such as unintentional injury, may be coded as maternal deaths due to the checkbox.

Discussion

This chapter examined the impact of the implementation of the 2003 revision of the U.S. Standard Certificate of Death on MMRs in the United States and related trends from 1999 through 2017. Results suggest that the implementation of the revised standard certificate, which included a question to determine pregnancy status (the pregnancy checkbox), was associated with an increased identification of maternal deaths. Averaging over the period 2003–2017, the checkbox resulted in an MMR increase of 9.6 deaths per 100,000 live births (95% CI: 8.6–10.6).

Impact of the Checkbox

The impact of the checkbox on MMRs was larger among older age groups, particularly ages 40 and over. A companion report that calculated maternal mortality rates for 2015–2016 with and without considering the pregnancy checkbox also found that the impact of the checkbox was largest for older age groups. In general, the MMRs in that report that did not consider the pregnancy checkbox (based only on information in the literal text) were similar to the estimated MMRs in this chapter, assuming that no states had adopted the checkbox. However, the estimated MMRs assuming that no states had adopted the checkbox tended to be somewhat higher than the MMRs reported in Hoyert et al. (e.g., predicted MMRs for 2015 and 2016 were 11.7 and 12.2, respectively, compared with 8.7 in Hoyert et al. [15]), with larger discrepancies among women aged 40 and over (e.g., predicted MMRs for 2015 and 2016 were 77.5 and 82.6, respectively, compared with 30.6 and 31.1 in Hoyert et al.). These reports used different methodologies to evaluate the impact of the checkbox. One potential reason for discrepancies may be that with the addition of the checkbox, certifiers may be less likely to record pregnancy-related information in the literal text fields. Consequently, recoding death records without considering the checkbox may result in lower MMRs than would have been identified had the checkbox never been implemented.

Prior studies have suggested that the pregnancy checkbox had a larger impact on MMRs among older women, likely resulting in overestimates [17]. However, other studies have suggested that the degree to which maternal deaths were undercounted prior to the implementation of the checkbox was larger for older women and teenagers. For example, a study in Maryland using data from 1993 through 2000 suggested that 58% of maternal deaths among women aged 40 and over and 50% among women under age 20 were not reported on the death certificate, in contrast to 38% among all women [11]. A study of Texas data after the implementation of the checkbox suggested that there were higher proportions of false positives and false negatives among women over 35 compared with women under 25 [24]. While these estimates are based on only two states and not generalizable to the entire United States, it suggests that among the oldest and youngest age groups, maternal deaths may have been disproportionately underestimated prior to the implementation of the checkbox, which could partly explain the larger impact of the checkbox seen among these age groups in this chapter. Additionally, prior studies indicate that there is likely a greater percentage of false positives among older women due to the pregnancy checkbox, inflating MMRs among older ages [4, 17, 24, 37]. Thus, part of the increase seen due to the implementation of the checkbox may be related to these false positives.

Differences by race and Hispanic origin also were seen in the impact of the checkbox. The impact was smallest for Hispanic women and largest for non-Hispanic black women. It is unclear whether maternal deaths among non-Hispanic black women were disproportionately missed prior to the implementation of the checkbox, whether there is a greater number of false positives among this group after the adoption of the revised standard certificate, or both. Some evidence suggests that false positives are more likely among non-Hispanic black women compared with non-Hispanic white women [37].

Consistent with prior reports, the impact of the checkbox on MMRs was greatest for nonspecific causes of maternal death [4, 13, 15], including maternal deaths due to other obstetric conditions not elsewhere classified (O95–O99), and a group of nonspecific causes of maternal death (O26.8, O95, O99.8). These causes of death are more likely the ones for which the checkbox may be the only indication of a current or recent pregnancy and where errors in the pregnancy checkbox would have the greatest impact, inflating MMRs related to these causes. Consequently, errors in the application of the checkbox (indicating a current or recent pregnancy when that is not the case) may lead to deaths due to cancer or infectious disease, for example, being coded to a maternal cause of death. A companion report that examined MMRs during 2015–2016 without considering the checkbox information found that heart conditions and cancer were the causes of death most frequently identified when death certificates were re-coded without considering the pregnancy checkbox. Because these causes of death are more common with increasing age, errors in the application of the checkbox have a disproportionate impact on MMRs among older women. Additionally, deaths due to nonmaternal causes of such as unintentional injury may erroneously receive one of these nonspecific codes if the pregnancy checkbox indicates a current or recent pregnancy, depending upon what information appears in part 1 or part 2 of the death certificate [15, 39, 40].

Trends

Maternal mortality rates were predicted under two alternative scenarios: (1) assuming that no states adopted the checkbox and (2) assuming that all states implemented the checkbox throughout the entire period. Under both scenarios, predicted MMRs did not change significantly from 1999 through 2017 (–0.03, 95% CI: –0.09–0.03; and 0.04, 95% CI: –0.07–0.15, respectively) after adjustment for age, race and Hispanic origin, and state. In a companion report, MMRs during 2015–2016 without considering the pregnancy checkbox were similar to those for 2000–2001, suggesting that in the absence of the checkbox, MMRs would not have increased over that time period. However, results presented here suggest differences in the estimated trends by subgroup and by cause of death. Predicted MMRs declined from 1999 through 2017 for non-Hispanic black women, Hispanic women, and women aged 20–24 and 30–34. Consistent with previous studies [4], predicted MMRs increased for non-Hispanic white women and women aged 40 and over. Importantly, this analysis cannot determine what the true change was in maternal mortality over this time period, as it is unclear how much of the impact of the checkbox was due to better identification of true maternal deaths and how much was potentially due to an increase in false positives.

Consistent with prior studies [4, 15, 16], there were differences by cause of death in estimated trends. Predicted MMRs declined for several direct causes of maternal death, including pregnancy with abortive outcomes (O00–O07); edema, proteinuria, and hypertensive disorders in pregnancy, childbirth and the puerperium (O10–O16); complications of labor and delivery (O60–O75); and complications predominantly related to the puerperium (O85–O92). Among all direct causes, excluding the nonspecific code O26.8, predicted MMRs declined by 0.17 each year (95% CI: –0.10– –0.01) assuming no checkbox and by 0.22 (95% CI: –0.30– –0.15) assuming that all states had adopted the checkbox. Conversely, predicted MMRs increased for several indirect and nonspecific causes of maternal death, including other specified pregnancy-related conditions (O26.8); late maternal deaths (O96–O97); and the group of nonspecific causes (O26.8, O95, O99.8). It is unclear to what extent these increases may be a consequence of nonmaternal deaths (e.g., deaths due to drug overdose or unintentional injury) being assigned one of these nonspecific or indirect cause-of-death codes due to the pregnancy checkbox being selected, possibly in error. The falsification tests suggested that the percentage of all deaths among reproductive-age women due to unintentional injuries, suicide, homicide, drug overdose, or unknown or ill-defined causes declined with the implementation of the checkbox. Small increases were observed among women for whom the pregnancy checkbox does not apply (under age 10 or 55–59), largely driven by increases in drug overdose deaths. This would suggest that a small percentage of nonmaternal deaths may be misclassified as maternal among women of reproductive age.

Misclassification

Based on prior research, death certificate data may both over- and underestimate maternal or pregnancy-associated deaths. Results presented in this chapter describe how MMRs may vary across a range of plausible values for Se and PVP. Studies that have conducted data linkages to evaluate the validity of the death certificate data in capturing maternal or pregnancy-associated deaths before the 2003 revision have suggested that as many as 40%–70% of pregnancies among decedents were historically not captured by death certificate data [8, 12, 22, 34, 36]. Similar studies conducted after the implementation of the checkbox have found that many maternal deaths have no evidence of current or recent pregnancy and that many current or recent pregnancies are not captured, with Se values (the proportion of true pregnancies among female decedents identified using death certificate data) ranging from 0.48 to 0.84 [13, 17–24, 33–35], and PVP values (the proportion of maternal deaths where a current or recent pregnancy is identified) ranging from 0.32 to 1.00 [20, 24, 41]. While national estimates of Se and PVP for identifying maternal deaths in death certificate data are not available, results from a recent study of four states suggest that Se (0.62) is slightly lower than PVP (0.68) [37]. If these values are similar across the United States, then overall MMRs may be slightly underestimated, with the number of false positives smaller than the number of false negatives. One potential limitation of these types of linkage studies is the lack of information on pregnancies that have not been documented in electronic medical records, or resulted in a live birth or fetal death, which would tend to deflate PVP values.

The degree of misclassification likely varies by many factors, including age, race and Hispanic origin, state, and cause of death. Because maternal deaths are a rare event, few studies have provided estimates of Se and PVP by subgroup. A study of Texas data after the implementation of the checkbox suggested that Se and PVP values were lower for women over age 35 than for women under 25 [24]. There were also differences by racial and ethnic group, with a smaller proportion of false negatives among non-Hispanic black and Hispanic women, and a higher proportion of false positives among non-Hispanic black and non-Hispanic white women [24]. However, severe data quality issues in that state [23, 24, 42] preclude those findings from being generalized to the United States. Other studies have also suggested that false positives are more likely among older age groups compared with younger age groups and among non-Hispanic black women compared with non-Hispanic white women [37]. Future studies providing more detail on Se and PVP by demographic subgroup across a wider array of states could facilitate a better understanding of the accuracy of MMRs and inform analyses adjusting for misclassification differentially by age, race and Hispanic origin, and other factors.

This analysis has several limitations. West Virginia did not adopt the revised standard certificate until mid-2017. Thus, estimates of the impact of the revision for West Virginia will be understated. California uses a question that is inconsistent with the 2003 standard certificate; it asks about pregnancy status in the past 12 months. Consequently, maternal deaths (during pregnancy or within 42 days) are likely underestimated in California, while late maternal deaths (pregnant within 43 days to 1 year) may be overstated given that checkbox-only deaths are coded to the late maternal category. Maryland, which was the only state to show a decline in MMRs with the implementation of the revised certificate, had a question prior to the revision that asked about pregnancy in the past year along with the corresponding date of delivery. It is possible that the decline in MMRs with the implementation of the revised standard certificate in Maryland is due to efforts in that state to identify maternal or pregnancy-associated deaths through data linkages and record reviews prior to implementing the revision. It is also possible that this decrease was due to chance, and no adjustments were made for multiple comparisons in this analysis. Because many states had some type of question about pregnancy status on the death certificate prior to the 2003 revision, the predicted MMRs assuming that no states had adopted the checkbox may be overestimated, as some of these states did have a pregnancy question prior to the revision.

Analyses adjusting for various error rates in the application of the checkbox on the death certificates only account for potential false positives, resulting in a likely underestimation of MMRs, as death certificate data often fail to capture many true maternal deaths. These analyses also assumed a constant error rate over time, which may not be accurate; they were based on error rates among women outside of reproductive age, which may not be comparable with the error rates among reproductive-age women. Adjustments for outcome misclassification, which account for both over- and underreporting of maternal deaths, likely provide better estimates of MMR values and trends. However, the true values for Se and PVP for the United States (and by subgroup or cause of death) are unknown, and thus these analyses are largely exploratory. It remains unknown to what extent the implementation of the pregnancy checkbox resulted in better ascertainment of maternal deaths (i.e., reductions in false negatives) and to what extent the checkbox may have increased false positives. Other data sources provide information about maternal or pregnancy-related mortality, such as the Pregnancy Mortality Surveillance System [6], data from maternal mortality review committees [20], and state- based quality-assurance projects [37]. These data sources, which rely on detailed record reviews or data linkages to verify recent pregnancy status, may not be subject to the same degree of misclassification as vital records data. Finally, there may have been other factors that changed simultaneously when states revised their death certificates, confounding the estimated impact of the checkbox. Specifically, the adoption of electronic death registration systems, the implementation of various quality-assurance processes (e.g., data linkages with birth and fetal death records), and the centralization of coding cause of death at NCHS. While an indicator for when coding was completely centralized (in 2011) was included in the models, many states had already relied on NCHS to code cause-of-death information prior to 2011. Specific information regarding what years various states were responsible for cause-of-death coding prior to 2011 is not available. State-specific estimates of the impact of the checkbox may be confounded by unmeasured factors that changed at the time of the revision, such as severe influenza seasons [43], rapid increases in drug overdose mortality [44], or loss of hospital-based obstetric services [45], among other potential factors. While higher-order trends (i.e., quadratic) were not apparent at the national level, it is possible that trends in MMRs in specific states before or after the revision were nonlinear, which could have biased estimated state-level impacts of the checkbox.

Conclusion

This chapter examines the impact of the staggered adoption of the 2003 revision of the standard death certificate on trends in maternal mortality in the United States from 1999 through 2017. Results suggest that the observed increases in MMRs during this time period were largely due to the staggered implementation of the checkbox, which increased identification of maternal deaths. Averaging over the period 2003–2017, the checkbox resulted in an MMR increase of 9.6 deaths per 100,000 live births (95% CI: 8.6–10.6). Estimated trends accounting for the implementation of the checkbox indicated that there were no significant changes in MMRs over time, although trends varied by maternal age, race and Hispanic origin, and cause of maternal death. Additionally, the misclassification of pregnancy status on the death certificate likely contributed to increasing trends among women aged 40 and over and among nonspecific causes of maternal death.

References

[1] Global Burden of Disease Maternal Mortality Collaborators. Global, regional, and national levels of maternal mortality, 1990–2015: A systematic analysis for the Global Burden of Disease Study 2015. *Lancet* 388(10053):1775–812. 2016.

[2] Hunt PH, Bueno de Mesquita J. *Reducing maternal mortality: The contribution of the right to the highest attainable standard of health*. 2010.

[3] World Health Organization. *Trends in maternal mortality: 1990 to 2015: Estimates by WHO, UNICEF, UNFPA, The World Bank Group and the United Nations Population Division*. 2015.

[4] MacDorman MF, Declercq E, Thoma ME. Trends in maternal mortality by sociodemographic characteristics and cause of death in

27 states and the District of Columbia. *Obstet Gynecol* 129(5):811–8. 2017.

[5] Neggers YH. Trends in maternal mortality in the United States. *Reprod Toxicol* 64:72–6. 2016.

[6] Petersen EE, Davis NL, Goodman D, Cox S, Mayes N, Johnston E, et al. Vital signs: Pregnancy-related deaths, United States, 2011–2015, and strategies for prevention, 13 states, 2013–2017. *MMWR Morb Mortal Wkly Rep* 68(18):423–9. 2019.

[7] Petersen EE, Davis NL, Goodman D, Cox S, Syverson C, Seed K, et al. Racial/ethnic disparities in pregnancy- related deaths—United States, 2007–2016. *MMWR Morb Mortal Wkly Rep* 68(35):762–5. 2019.

[8] Horon IL, Cheng D. Effectiveness of pregnancy check boxes on death certificates in identifying pregnancy- associated mortality. *Public Health Rep* 126(2):195– 200. 2011.

[9] MacKay AP, Berg CJ, Duran C, Chang J, Rosenberg H. An assessment of pregnancy-related mortality in the United States. *Paediatr Perinat Epidemiol* 19(3):206– 14. 2005.

[10] Hoyert DL, Danel I, Tully P. Maternal mortality, United States and Canada, 1982–1997. Birth 27(1):4–11. 2000.

[11] Horon IL. Underreporting of maternal deaths on death certificates and the magnitude of the problem of maternal mortality. *Am J Public Health* 95(3):478–82. 2005.

[12] Horon IL, Cheng D. Enhanced surveillance for pregnancy-associated mortality—Maryland, 1993– 1998. *JAMA* 285(11):1455–9. 2001.

[13] Creanga AA. Maternal mortality in the United States: A review of contemporary data and their limitations. *Clin Obstet Gynecol* 61(2):296–306. 2018.

[14] MacDorman MF, Declercq E, Cabral H, Morton C. Recent increases in the U.S. maternal mortality rate: Disentangling trends from measurement issues. *Obstet Gynecol* 128(3):447–55. 2016.

[15] Hoyert DL, Uddin SFG, Miniño AM. Maternal mortality evaluation: Impact of the inclusion of a pregnancy status checkbox item on death

certificates. *National Vital Statistics Reports*; vol 69 no 2. Hyattsville, MD: National Center for Health Statistics. 2019.

[16] Joseph KS, Lisonkova S, Muraca GM, Razaz N, Sabr Y, Mehrabadi A, Schisterman EF. Factors underlying the temporal increase in maternal mortality in the United States. *Obstet Gynecol* 129(1):91–100. 2017.

[17] Davis NL, Hoyert DL, Goodman DA, Hirai AH, Callaghan WM. Contribution of maternal age and pregnancy checkbox on maternal mortality ratios in the United States, 1978–2012. *Am J Obstet Gynecol* 217(3):352. e1–7. 2017.

[18] Nelson DB, Moniz MH, Davis MM. Population- level factors associated with maternal mortality in the United States, 1997–2012. *BMC Public Health* 18(1):1007. 2018.

[19] Daymude AEC, Catalano A, Goodman D. Checking the pregnancy checkbox: Evaluation of a four-state quality assurance pilot. *Birth* 46(4):648–55. 2019.

[20] *Building U.S. Capacity to Review and Prevent Maternal Deaths Project Team.* Report from nine maternal mortality review committees. 2018.

[21] St Pierre A, Zaharatos J, Goodman D, Callaghan WM. Challenges and opportunities in identifying, reviewing, and preventing maternal deaths. *Obstet Gynecol* 131(1):138–42. 2018.

[22] Mitchell C, Lawton E, Morton C, McCain C, Holtby S, Main E. California pregnancy-associated mortality review: Mixed methods approach for improved case identification, cause of death analyses and translation of findings. *Matern Child Health J* 18(3):518–26. 2014.

[23] MacDorman MF, Declercq E, Thoma ME. Trends in Texas maternal mortality by maternal age, race/ ethnicity, and cause of death, 2006–2015. *Birth* 45(2):169–77. 2018.

[24] Baeva S, Saxton DL, Ruggiero K, Kormondy ML, Hollier LM, Hellerstedt J, et al. Identifying maternal deaths in Texas using an enhanced method, 2012. *Obstet Gynecol* 131(5):762–9. 2018.

[25] National Center for Health Statistics. *National Vital Statistics System: Birth data.* Available from: https://www.cdc.gov/nchs/nvss/births.htm.

[26] Say L, Chou D, Gemmill A, Tunçalp Ö, Moller AB, Daniels J, et al. Global causes of maternal death: A WHO systematic analysis. *Lancet Glob Health* 2(6):e323–33. 2014.

[27] Oldenburg CE, Moscoe E, Bärnighausen T. Regression discontinuity for causal effect estimation in epidemiology. *Curr Epidemiol Rep* 3:233–41. 2016.

[28] Bor J, Moscoe E, Mutevedzi P, Newell ML, Bärnighausen T. Regression discontinuity designs in epidemiology: Causal inference without randomized trials. *Epidemiology* 25(5):729–37. 2014.

[29] Moscoe E, Bor J, Bärnighausen T. Regression discontinuity designs are underutilized in medicine, epidemiology, and public health: A review of current and best practice. *J Clin Epidemiol* 68(2):122–33. 2015.

[30] Ventura SJ. The U.S. National Vital Statistics System: transitioning into the 21st century, 1990–2017. National Center for Health Statistics. *Vital Health Stat* 1(62). 2018.

[31] Lash TL, Fox MP, Fink AK. Applying quantitative bias analysis to epidemiologic data. In: Gail M, Samet JM, Tsiatis A, Wong W, editors. *Statistics for biology and health.* New York, NY: Springer. 2009.

[32] Rothman KJ, Greenland S, Lash TL. *Modern epidemiology*. 3rd ed. Philadelphia, PA: Lippincott Williams & Wilkins. 2008.

[33] Saucedo M, Bouvier-Colle MH, Chantry AA, Lamarche- Vadel A, Rey G, Deneux-Tharaux C. Pitfalls of national routine death statistics for maternal mortality study. *Paediatr Perinat Epidemiol* 28(6):479–88. 2014.

[34] Tran T, Roberson E, Borstell J, Hoyert DL. Evaluation of pregnancy mortality in Louisiana using enhanced linkage and different indicators defined by WHO and CDC/ACOG: Challenging and practical issues. *Matern Child Health J* 15(7):955–63. 2011.

[35] Tennessee Department of Health. *Tennessee maternal mortality: Review of 2017 maternal deaths.* 2017.

[36] California Department of Public Health. *The California pregnancy-associated mortality review: Report from 2002 to 2007 maternal death reviews.* 2018.

[37] Catalano A, Davis NL, Petersen EE, Harrison C, Kieltyka L, You M, et al. Pregnant? Validity of the pregnancy checkbox on death certificates in four states, and characteristics associated with pregnancy checkbox errors. *Am J Obstet Gynecol.* S0002–9378(19)31222–0. 2019.

[38] Deneux-Tharaux C, Berg C, Bouvier-Colle MH, Gissler M, Harper M, Nannini A, et al. Underreporting of pregnancy-related mortality in the United States and Europe. *Obstet Gynecol* 106(4):684–92. 2005.

[39] National Center for Health Statistics. *Instructions for classifying underlying and multiple causes of death, ICD–10. 2017.*

[40] Anderson RN. Maternal deaths in the National Vital Statistics System. In: *2019 Proceedings of the National Center for Health Statistics Board of Scientific Counselors*. Hyattsville, MD: National Center for Health Statistics. 2019.

[41] Building U.S. Capacity to Review and Prevent Maternal Deaths Project Team. *Report from maternal mortality review committees: A view into their critical role*. 2017.

[42] Koch AR, Lightner S, Geller SE. Identifying maternal deaths in Texas using an enhanced method, 2012. *Obstet Gynecol* 132(2):520–1. 2018.

[43] Callaghan WM, Creanga AA, Jamieson DJ. Pregnancy- related mortality resulting from influenza in the United States during the 2009–2010 pandemic. *Obstet Gynecol* 126(3):486–90. 2015.

[44] Goldman-Mellor S, Margerison CE. Maternal drug- related death and suicide are leading causes of post-partum death in California. *Am J Obstet Gynecol* 221(15):489.e1–9. 2019.

[45] Kozhimannil KB, Hung P, Henning-Smith C, Casey MM, Prasad S. Association between loss of hospital-based obstetric services and birth outcomes in rural counties in the United States. *JAMA* 319(12):1239–47. 2018.

Table 1. Average change in maternal mortality rates associated with the pregnancy checkbox implementation, by age and race and Hispanic origin: United States, 2003–2017

Characteristic	Change in maternal mortality rate (95% CI)
Overall	9.6 (8.6 – 10.6)
Age group	
Under 15	14.5 (–10.3 – 39.3)
15–19	3.7 (1.7 – 5.7)
20–24	5.6 (4.1 – 7.1)
25–29	5.4 (3.8 – 7.1)
30–34	6.0 (3.9 – 8.0)
35–39	13.9 (9.7 – 18.0)
40 and over	145.3 (127.6 – 163.1)
Race and Hispanic origin	
Non-Hispanic white	8.6 (7.5 – 9.7)
Non-Hispanic black	19.6 (15.3 – 24.0)
Non-Hispanic other	7.1 (4.2 – 10.0)
Hispanic	6.2 (4.3 – 8.1)
Prerevision pregnancy question	
No	9.8 (8.7 – 10.9)
Yes	8.1 (6.8 – 9.4)
Centralized cause-of-death coding	
No (before 2011)	9.0 (8.0 – 10.0)
Yes (2011–2017)	10.9 (9.5 – 12.2)

Note: CI is confidence interval.

Source: NCHS, National Vital Statistics System, 1999–2017.

Table 2. Trends in predicted maternal mortality rates, by age and race and Hispanic origin: United States, 1999–2017

Characteristic	Average annual change in maternal mortality rate			
	No checkbox (95% CI)	*p*	All checkbox (95% CI)	*p*
Overall	0.0 (–0.1 – 0.0)	0.307	0.0 (– 0.1 – 0.2)	0.459
Age group				
Under 15	0.4 (–0.8 – 1.5)	0.519	1.7 (–1.9 – 5.3)	0.359
15–19	0.0 (–0.1 – 0.1)	0.616	0.1 (–0.1 – 0.3)	0.538
20–24	– 0.1 (–0.2 – 0.0)	0.001	–0.2 (–0.4 – –0.1)	0.008
25–29	– 0.1 (– 0.2 – 0.0)	0.057	– 0.1 (–0.3 – 0.0)	0.116
30–34	– 0.2 (– 0.3 – –0.1)	0.002	– 0.3 (–0.5 – –0.1)	0.013
35–39	– 0.1 (– 0.3 – 0.1)	0.425	– 0.1 (–0.5 – 0.3)	0.552
40 and over	2.5 (1.8 – 3.3)	Less than 0.001	7.7 (6.1 – 9.4)	Less than 0.001
Race and Hispanic origin				
Non-Hispanic white	0.1 (0.1 – 0.2)	Less than 0.001	0.3 (0.2 – 0.5)	Less than 0.001
Non-Hispanic black	– 0.3 (– 0.6 – –0.1)	0.004	– 0.4 (–0.9 – 0.0)	0.072
Non-Hispanic other	– 0.1 (– 0.3 – 0.0)	0.104	– 0.2 (–0.4 – 0.1)	0.280
Hispanic	– 0.3 (– 0.3 – –0.2)	Less than 0.001	– 0.4 (–0.6 – –0.2)	Less than 0.001

Note: CI is confidence interval.

Source: NCHS, National Vital Statistics System, 1999–2017.

Table 3. Estimated impact of the pregnancy checkbox on cause-specific maternal mortality rates: United States, 2003–2017

Cause of maternal death	Average change in maternal mortality rate (95% CI)
Direct causes	5.2 (4.4 – 6.1)
Direct causes excluding O26.8	2.0 (1.3 – 2.7)
Alternative grouping of direct causes (A34,O00–O92)	4.8 (4.0 – 5.6)
Alternative grouping of direct causes (A34,O00–O95)	5.6 (4.8 – 6.5)
O00–O07: Pregnancy with abortive outcomes	0.2 (0.0 – 0.5)
O10–O16: Edema, proteinuria and hypertensive disorders in pregnancy, childbirth and the puerperium	0.4 (0.0 – 0.7)
O20–O29: Other maternal disorders predominantly related to pregnancy	3.5 (3.1 – 4.0)
O26.6: Liver disorders in pregnancy, childbirth and the puerperium	0.5 (0.3 – 0.7)
O26.8: Other specified pregnancy-related conditions	2.6 (2.2 – 2.9)

Cause of maternal death	Average change in maternal mortality rate (95% CI)
O20–O29: Other maternal disorders predominantly related to pregnancy, excluding O26.8	1.0 (0.8 – 1.3)
O30–O48: Maternal care related to the fetus and amniotic cavity and possible delivery problems	0.3 (0.0 – 0.5)
O60–O75: Complications of labor and delivery	0.2 (– 0.1 – 0.5)
O85–O92: Complications predominantly related to the puerperium	0.4 (0.0 – 0.8)
Indirect causes	4.6 (4.1 – 5.1)
Alternative grouping of indirect causes (O98–O99)	4.2 (3.7 – 4.7)
O95–O99: Other obstetric conditions not elsewhere classified (including late maternal deaths)	8.3 (7.6 – 9.0)
O95,O98–O99: Other obstetric conditions not elsewhere classified (excluding late maternal deaths)	5.1 (4.6 – 5.6)
O99.3: Mental disorders and diseases of the nervous system complicating pregnancy, childbirth and the puerperium	0.2 (0.1 – 0.3)
O99.4: Diseases of the circulatory system complicating pregnancy, childbirth and the puerperium	1.2 (0.9 – 1.4)
O99.5: Diseases of the respiratory system complicating pregnancy, childbirth and the puerperium	0.4 (0.2 – 0.6)
O99.8: Other specified diseases and conditions complicating pregnancy, childbirth and the puerperium	2.3 (1.9 – 2.6)
O96–O97: Late maternal deaths	3.5 (3.1 – 3.9)
Nonspecific causes (O26.8,O95,O99.8)	5.6 (5.1 – 6.1)

Notes: CI is confidence interval. Direct and indirect causes of maternal death from Say et al.; see reference 26 in this chapter. Alternative grouping of direct causes of maternal death (A34,O00–O92) and indirect causes (O98–O99) from MacDorman et al.; see reference 4 in this chapter. Alternative grouping of direct causes of maternal death (A34,O00–O95) from Hoyert et al.; see reference 15 in this chapter.

Source: NCHS, National Vital Statistics System, 1999–2017.

Table 4. Estimated trends in predicted maternal mortality rates, by cause of death: United States, 1999–2017

Average annual change in maternal mortality rate				
Cause of maternal death	No checkbox (95% CI)	*p*	All checkbox (95% CI)	*p*
Direct causes	– 0.05 (–0.10 – 0.01)	0.083	– 0.08 (–0.17 – 0.01)	0.099
Direct causes excluding O26.8	– 0.17 (–0.22 – –0.12)	Less than 0.001	– 0.22 (–0.30 – – 0.15)	Less than 0.001
Alternative grouping of direct causes (A34,O00–O92)	0.00 (–0.05 – 0.06)	0.950	0.00 (–0.08 – 0.09)	0.953

Table 4. (Continued)

Average annual change in maternal mortality rate				
Cause of maternal death	No checkbox (95% CI)	*p*	All checkbox (95% CI)	*p*
Alternative grouping of direct causes (A34,O00–O95)	– 0.03 (–0.09 – 0.02)	0.228	– 0.05 (–0.15 – 0.04)	0.242
O00–O07: Pregnancy with abortive outcomes	– 0.03 (–0.05 – –0.02)	Less than 0.001	– 0.05 (–0.07 – – 0.02)	0.001
O10–O16: Edema, proteinuria and hypertensive disorders in pregnancy, childbirth and the puerperium	– 0.03 (–0.05 – 0.00)	0.019	– 0.04 (–0.07 – 0.00)	0.045
O20–O29: Other maternal disorders predominantly related to pregnancy	0.09 (0.06 – 0.12)	Less than 0.001	0.26 (0.21 – 0.31)	Less than 0.001
O26.6: Liver disorders in pregnancy, childbirth and the puerperium	0.00 (0.00 – 0.01)	0.244	0.02 (–0.01 – 0.04)	0.145
O26.8: Other specified pregnancy-related conditions (pregnancy-related exhaustion and fatigue, peripheral neuritis or renal disease)	0.08 (0.05 – 0.10)	Less than 0.001	0.25 (0.21 – 0.29)	Less than 0.001
O20–O29: Other maternal disorders predominantly related to pregnancy, excluding O26.8	0.00 (–0.01 – 0.02)	0.575	0.01 (–0.02 – 0.04)	0.554
O30–O48: Maternal care related to the fetus and amniotic cavity and possible delivery problems	– 0.01 (–0.03 – 0.00)	0.039	– 0.02 (–0.05 – 0.00)	0.094
O60–O75: Complications of labor and delivery	– 0.06 (–0.08 – –0.04)	Less than 0.001	– 0.08 (–0.11 – – 0.04)	Less than 0.001
O85–O92: Complications predominantly related to the puerperium	– 0.03 (–0.06 – 0.00)	0.021	– 0.04 (–0.08 – 0.00)	0.045
Indirect causes	0.03 (0.01 – 0.05)	0.008	0.10 (0.04 – 0.16)	0.002
Alternative grouping of indirect causes (O98–O99)	0.02 (0.00 – 0.04)	0.037	0.07 (0.01 – 0.14)	0.019

Average annual change in maternal mortality rate				
Cause of maternal death	No checkbox (95% CI)	*p*	All checkbox (95% CI)	*p*
O95–O99: Other obstetric conditions not elsewhere classified (including late maternal deaths)	0.13 (0.09 – 0.16)	Less than 0.001	0.39 (0.31 – 0.46)	Less than 0.001
O95,O98–O99: Other obstetric conditions not elsewhere classified (excluding late maternal deaths)	0.00 (–0.02 – 0.02)	0.895	0.00 (–0.07 – 0.08)	0.897
O99.3: Mental disorders and diseases of the nervous system complicating pregnancy, childbirth and the puerperium	0.00 (0.00 – 0.01)	0.108	0.02 (0.01 – 0.03)	0.004
O99.4: Diseases of the circulatory system complicating pregnancy, childbirth and the puerperium	0.00 (–0.01 – 0.02)	0.538	0.01 (–0.02 – 0.04)	0.514
O99.5: Diseases of the respiratory system complicating pregnancy, childbirth and the puerperium	0.00 (–0.01 – 0.00)	0.089	– 0.02 (–0.04 – 0.01)	0.225
O99.8: Other specified diseases and conditions complicating pregnancy, childbirth and the puerperium	0.01 (0.00 – 0.02)	0.141	0.04 (–0.01 – 0.08)	0.095
O96–O97: Late maternal deaths	0.12 (0.09 – 0.15)	Less than 0.001	0.34 (0.29 – 0.39)	Less than 0.001
Nonspecific causes (O26.8,O95,O99.8)	0.06 (0.04 – 0.09)	Less than 0.001	0.23 (0.17 – 0.30)	Less than 0.001

Notes: CI is confidence interval. Models were adjusted for age group, race and Hispanic origin, and state of occurrence, and included interactions between year and age and year and race and Hispanic origin. Models for O99.3 did not include state of occurrence. Direct and indirect causes of maternal death from Say et al.; see reference 26 in this chapter. Alternative grouping of direct causes of maternal death (A34,O00–O92) and indirect causes (O98–O99) from MacDorman et al.; see reference 4 in this chapter. Alternative grouping of direct causes of maternal death (A34,O00–O95) from Hoyert et al.; see reference 15 in this chapter.

Source: NCHS, National Vital Statistics System, 1999–2017.

Table 5. Estimated average change in the percentage of all deaths due to nonmaternal causes of death associated with the implementation of the revised standard death certificate, by age: United States, 2003–2017

Cause of death	Change in percentage of all deaths			
	15–44 years (95% CI)	*p*	Under 10 years or 55–59 (95% CI)	*p*
Unintentional injury (V01–X59,Y85–86)	–0.14 (–0.43 – 0.15)	0.344	0.15 (0.00 – 0.29)	0.047
Suicide (*U03,X60–X84,Y87.0)	–0.04 (–0.22 – 0.13)	0.635	0.04 (–0.03 – 0.10)	0.304
Drug overdose (X40–X44, X60–X64, X85, Y10–Y14)	0.86 (0.63 – 1.09)	Less than 0.001	0.37 (0.28 – 0.46)	Less than 0.001
Homicide (*U01–*U02,X85–Y09,Y87.1)	–0.10 (–0.24 – 0.04)	0.159	0.03 (–0.02 – 0.09)	0.253
Unknown (R99)	–0.40 (–0.50 – –0.31)	Less than 0.001	–0.03 (–0.10 – 0.04)	0.445
All	–0.53 (–0.85 – –0.20)	0.001	0.21 (0.03 – 0.39)	0.020

Notes: CI is confidence interval. Models were adjusted for age group, race and Hispanic origin, and state of occurrence, and included interactions between year and age and year and race and Hispanic origin.

Source: CDC/NCHS, National Vital Statistics System, 1999–2017.

Appendix I. Supplemental Tables and Details of Adjustments to Maternal Mortality Ratios for Misclassification

Table A-I displays the percentage of records where one of the pregnancy checkboxes was selected (either currently pregnant, pregnant within 42 days, or pregnant 43 days to 1 year) among women of ages where pregnancy would be implausible (under age 10 or 55 and over) by state of occurrence.

Table A-I. Percentage of deaths among female decedents under 10 years or 55 and over where one of the pregnancy checkboxes was selected, by state of occurrence: 2003–2013

	Under 10		**55 and over**		
State	Percent	*N*	Percent	*N*	Row total percent
Arizona	0.00	1,171	0.03	82,287	0.03
Arkansas	0.00	985	0.01	75,536	0.01
California	0.19	16,684	0.13	1,144,060	0.14
Connecticut	0.00	1,026	0.02	127,400	0.02
Delaware	0.00	383	0.01	23,875	0.01
District of Columbia	0.10	963	0.05	20,136	0.06
Florida	0.00	7,749	0.00	669,133	0.00
Georgia	0.00	3,184	0.02	186,774	0.02
Idaho	0.00	731	0.00	52,937	0.00
Illinois	0.03	3,420	0.02	274,518	0.02
Indiana	0.00	2,052	0.02	158,774	0.02
Iowa	0.00	278	0.01	40,410	0.01
Kansas	0.00	1,215	0.00	100,248	0.00
Kentucky	0.00	751	0.08	74,324	0.07
Louisiana	0.00	599	0.02	36,154	0.02
Maine	0.00	195	0.00	23,942	0.00
Michigan	0.10	4,848	0.08	393,437	0.08
Minnesota	0.00	624	0.01	56,209	0.01
Mississippi	0.00	351	0.00	25,082	0.00
Missouri	0.00	1,308	0.02	103,928	0.02
Montana	0.00	430	0.00	42,063	0.00
Nebraska	0.00	793	0.00	65,048	0.00
Nevada	0.00	668	0.04	48,836	0.04
New Hampshire	0.00	331	0.06	48,203	0.06
New Jersey	0.45	2,648	0.11	329,523	0.12
New Mexico	0.00	695	0.02	50,912	0.02
New York city	0.00	4,069	0.01	270,083	0.01
New York state	0.05	4,173	0.08	502,104	0.08
North Dakota	0.00	186	0.34	17,417	0.34
Ohio	0.00	4,275	0.02	354,857	0.02
Oklahoma	0.04	2,299	0.09	154,725	0.09
Oregon	0.00	1,205	0.01	116,620	0.01
Pennsylvania	0.00	1,125	0.00	121,313	0.00

Table A-I. (Continued)

	Under 10		55 and over		
State	Percent	*N*	Percent	*N*	Row total percent
Rhode Island	0.00	354	0.06	38,025	0.06
South Carolina	0.00	2,163	0.00	155,152	0.00
South Dakota	0.00	492	0.00	32,372	0.00
Tennessee	0.00	763	0.07	57,115	0.07
Texas	0.06	10,931	0.05	571,070	0.05
Utah	0.21	1,424	0.07	56,793	0.07
Vermont	0.00	84	0.02	14,747	0.02
Washington	0.00	2,335	0.00	215,329	0.00
Wisconsin	0.00	220	0.01	22,968	0.01
Wyoming	0.00	165	0.00	16,887	0.00

Notes: Beginning in 2014, records indicating current or recent pregnancy among female decedents under 10 or 55 and over were recoded to "Not Applicable." States that adopted the revised standard certificate in 2014 or later are therefore not shown.

Source: NCHS, National Vital Statistics System, 2003–2013.

Table A-II displays differences in maternal mortality rates associated with the implementation of the checkbox by state of occurrence.

Table A-II. Change in maternal mortality rates associated with the pregnancy checkbox implementation, by state of occurrence

State	Change in maternal mortality rate (95% CI)
Alabama	29.0 (18.4 – 39.7)
Alaska	4.0 (–8.7 – 16.7)
Arizona	10.2 (2.2 – 18.1)
Arkansas	15.7 (1.0 – 30.4)
California	9.9 (5.2 – 14.7)
Colorado	2.0 (–4.8 – 8.8)
Connecticut	5.7 (–0.6 – 12.0)
Delaware	19.0 (–15.5 – 53.5)
District of Columbia	2.3 (–9.9 – 14.6)
Florida	9.3 (4.8 – 13.7)
Georgia	3.2 (–2.4 – 8.7)
Hawaii	–6.4 (–22.3 – 9.5)
Idaho	23.9 (4.7 – 43.2)
Illinois	17.9 (10.6 – 25.1)
Indiana	20.4 (14.3 – 26.5)
Iowa	9.5 (–1.7 – 20.7)

State	Change in maternal mortality rate (95% CI)
Kansas	14.0 (4.3 – 23.8)
Kentucky	11.6 (0.6 – 22.7)
Louisiana	38.2 (28.4 – 48.0)
Maine	6.9 (–13.5 – 27.3)
Maryland	–7.8 (–13.3 – –2.4)
Massachusetts	2.4 (–1.6 – 6.5)
Michigan	29.9 (20.4 – 39.3)
Minnesota	1.5 (–6.2 – 9.2)
Mississippi	–10.0 (–21.4 – 1.5)
Missouri	6.5 (–3.9 – 16.9)
Montana	0.4 (–24.2 – 25.0)
Nebraska	–2.6 (–16.8 – 11.7)
Nevada	–1.3 (–12.7 – 10.0)
New Hampshire	5.3 (–12.9 – 23.4)
New Jersey	16.1 (11.0 – 21.1)
New Mexico	15.7 (–5.9 – 37.2)
New York City	9.3 (2.7 – 15.9)
New York State[1]	6.6 (1.8 – 11.3)
North Carolina	9.5 (5.0 – 14.1)
North Dakota	25.3 (–14.3 – 64.9)
Ohio	19.6 (12.7 – 26.4)
Oklahoma	29.9 (16.0 – 43.8)
Oregon	5.1 (–3.7 – 13.9)
Pennsylvania	– 2.4 (–8.4 – 3.6)
Rhode Island	–0.8 (–13.5 – 11.8)
South Carolina	18.3 (9.8 – 26.7)
South Dakota	14.8 (–7.1 – 36.7)
Tennessee	18.8 (11.2 – 26.3)
Texas	12.5 (8.8 – 16.1)
Utah	10.9 (0.1 – 21.6)
Vermont	4.4 (–16.6 – 25.4)
Virginia	7.4 (2.5 – 12.3)
Washington	3.7 (–2.3 – 9.6)
West Virginia	4.6 (–17.4 – 26.6)
Wisconsin	–4.8 (–12.9 – 3.2)
Wyoming	84.4 (–22.5 – 191.3)

[1]Excludes New York City. NOTE: CI is confidence interval.

Source: NCHS, National Vital Statistics System, 1999–2017.

Table A-III displays the observed maternal mortality rates (MMRs), predicted MMRs assuming that no states had adopted the checkbox during this time period, and predicted MMRs assuming that all states had adopted the checkbox during the entire time period.

Table A-III. Observed and predicted maternal mortality rates: United States, 1999–2017

Year	Maternal mortality rate	Predicted maternal mortality rate, no checkbox	Predicted maternal mortality rate, all checkbox
1999	9.9 (8.9 – 10.9)	10.3 (7.4 – 13.2)	21.2 (11.2 – 31.2)
2000	9.8 (8.8 – 10.8)	10.1 (7.2 – 13.0)	20.8 (11.6 – 30.0)
2001	9.9 (8.9 – 10.9)	10.0 (7.3 – 12.7)	20.3 (11.5 – 29.1)
2002	8.9 (8.0 – 9.8)	9.8 (7.3 – 12.3)	19.8 (12.0 – 27.6)
2003	12.1 (11.0 – 13.2)	9.7 (7.2 – 12.2)	19.5 (12.4 – 26.6)
2004	13.1 (12.0 – 14.2)	9.7 (7.2 – 12.2)	19.2 (12.7 – 25.7)
2005	15.1 (13.9 – 16.3)	9.6 (7.1 – 12.1)	19.0 (12.5 – 25.5)
2006	13.3 (12.2 – 14.4)	9.7 (7.0 – 12.4)	18.7 (12.8 – 24.6)
2007	12.7 (11.6 – 13.8)	9.7 (6.8 – 12.6)	18.6 (13.1 – 24.1)
2008	15.5 (14.3 – 16.7)	9.8 (6.7 – 12.9)	18.7 (13.4 – 24.0)
2009	16.6 (15.4 – 17.8)	9.9 (6.6 – 13.2)	18.9 (14.2 – 23.6)
2010	16.9 (15.6 – 18.2)	10.1 (6.2 – 14.0)	19.2 (14.9 – 23.5)
2011	19.3 (17.9 – 20.7)	10.4 (6.1 – 14.7)	19.6 (14.9 – 24.3)
2012	19.9 (18.5 – 21.3)	10.6 (5.9 – 15.3)	19.9 (15.2 – 24.6)
2013	22.0 (20.5 – 23.5)	10.9 (5.6 – 16.2)	20.5 (16.2 – 24.8)
2014	21.5 (20.1 – 22.9)	11.3 (5.8 – 16.8)	20.9 (16.2 – 25.6)
2015	20.9 (19.5 – 22.3)	11.7 (6.2 – 17.2)	21.7 (16.6 – 26.8)
2016	21.8 (20.3 – 23.3)	12.2 (6.5 – 17.9)	22.4 (16.9 – 27.9)
2017	21.6 (20.1 – 23.1)	12.8 (6.5 – 19.1)	23.5 (17.4 – 29.6)

Note: Models were adjusted for age group, race and Hispanic origin, and state of occurrence, and included interactions between these factors and year as well as revision status.

Source: NCHS, National Vital Statistics System, 1999–2017.

Table A-IV displays the predicted MMRs assuming that no states had adopted the checkbox during this time period, and predicted MMRs assuming that all states had adopted the checkbox during the entire time period by varying degrees of outcome misclassification.

Table A-IV. Predicted maternal mortality rates, adjusted for outcome misclassification: United States, 1999 and 2017

Levels of outcome misclassification, by sensitivity and predictive value positive		**Predicted maternal mortality rate assuming no states had adopted the checkbox**		**Predicted maternal mortality rate assuming all states had adopted the checkbox**	
Sensitivity	Predictive value positive	1999	2017	1999	2017
0.3	0.5	17.1	21.4	35.3	39.2
0.3	0.6	20.5	25.6	42.4	47.1
0.3	0.7	24.0	29.9	49.5	54.9
0.3	0.8	27.4	34.2	56.6	62.8
0.3	0.9	30.8	38.5	63.6	70.6
0.4	0.5	12.8	16.0	26.5	29.4
0.4	0.6	15.4	19.2	31.8	35.3
0.4	0.7	18.0	22.4	37.1	41.2
0.4	0.8	20.5	25.6	42.4	47.1
0.4	0.9	23.1	28.8	47.7	52.9
0.5	0.5	10.3	12.8	21.2	23.5
0.5	0.6	12.3	15.4	25.4	28.2
0.5	0.7	14.4	17.9	29.7	32.9
0.5	0.8	16.4	20.5	33.9	37.7
0.5	0.9	18.5	23.1	38.2	42.4
0.6	0.5	8.6	10.7	17.7	19.6
0.6	0.6	10.3	12.8	21.2	23.5
0.6	0.7	12.0	15.0	24.7	27.5
0.6	0.8	13.7	17.1	28.3	31.4
0.6	0.9	15.4	19.2	31.8	35.3
0.7	0.5	7.3	9.2	15.1	16.8
0.7	0.6	8.8	11.0	18.2	20.2
0.7	0.7	10.3	12.8	21.2	23.5
0.7	0.8	11.7	14.7	24.2	26.9
0.7	0.9	13.2	16.5	27.3	30.3
0.8	0.5	6.4	8.0	13.3	14.7
0.8	0.6	7.7	9.6	15.9	17.6
0.8	0.7	9.0	11.2	18.6	20.6
0.8	0.8	10.3	12.8	21.2	23.5
0.8	0.9	11.6	14.4	23.9	26.5
0.9	0.5	5.7	7.1	11.8	13.1
0.9	0.6	6.8	8.5	14.1	15.7
0.9	0.7	8.0	10.0	16.5	18.3

Table A-IV. (Continued)

Levels of outcome misclassification, by sensitivity and predictive value positive		Predicted maternal mortality rate assuming no states had adopted the checkbox		Predicted maternal mortality rate assuming all states had adopted the checkbox	
Sensitivity	Predictive value positive	1999	2017	1999	2017
0.9	0.8	9.1	11.4	18.9	20.9
0.9	0.9	10.3	12.8	21.2	23.5

Note: Sensitivity refers to the proportion of true maternal deaths captured by death certificate data. Predictive value positive refers to the proportion of maternal deaths identified in death certificate data that are true maternal deaths.

Source: NCHS, National Vital Statistics System, 1999–2017.

Table A-V. Comparison of pregnancy status on death certificates with pregnancy status assessed by a gold standard measure

Death certificate			
Gold standard	Yes	No	Total
Yes	a	b	T_y
No	c	d	T_n
Total	D_y	D_n	Total number

Note: The gold standard is based on prior analyses of the validity of death certificate data in ascertaining maternal deaths, which rely on linkages of death certificates with birth certificate, fetal death certificate, and electronic medical record data to determine whether a female decedent was currently or recently pregnant.

Table A-V displays how death certificate data compare with gold standard data, where T_y is the true number of maternal deaths, and T_n is the number of nonmaternal deaths, while D_y is the number of maternal deaths as indicated by death certificate data, and D_n is the number of nonmaternal deaths.

Sensitivity (Se) is the proportion of true maternal deaths classified as maternal deaths on the death certificate. Predictive value positive (PVP) is the proportion of maternal deaths in mortality data that are truly maternal deaths. The proportion of maternal deaths from death certificate data that are false positives (FP) is 1 – *PVP*, corresponding to the proportion of maternal deaths with no evidence of current or recent pregnancy. Using these values, the true number of maternal deaths corrected for misclassification, T_y, can be calculated as follows:

$$Se = \frac{a}{T_y} \quad (1)$$

Therefore,

$$a = Se \bullet T_y \quad (2)$$

Additionally,

$$PVP = \frac{a}{D_y} \quad (3)$$

$$FP = (1 - PVP) = \frac{c}{D_y} \quad (4)$$

Therefore,

$$c = (1 - PVP) \bullet D_y \quad (5)$$

T_y is unknown, while D_y is observed, and values for Se and PVP are estimated from prior studies.

$$D_y = a + c = Se \bullet T_y + (1 - PVP) \bullet D_y \tag{6}$$

The following formula can then be used to calculate T_y from Se, PVP, and D_y:

$$T_y = \frac{D_y - (1 - PVP) \bullet D_y}{Se} = \frac{D_y \bullet PVP}{Se} \tag{7}$$

TECHNICAL NOTES

Cause-of-Death Classification

Mortality statistics are compiled in accordance with World Health Organization (WHO) regulations specifying that WHO member nations classify and code causes of death in accordance with the current revision of the *International Statistical Classification of Diseases and Related Health Problems* (ICD). ICD provides the basic guidance used in virtually all countries to code and classify causes of death. It provides not only disease, injury, and poisoning categories, but also the rules used to select the single underlying cause of death for tabulation from the conditions reported on the death certificate, as well as definitions, tabulation lists, the format of the death certificate, and regulations on use of the classification. Causes of death for data presented in this chapter were coded according to ICD guidelines described in annual issues of the National Center for Health Statistics instruction manuals (39).

APPENDIX II. SUPPLEMENTAL FIGURES

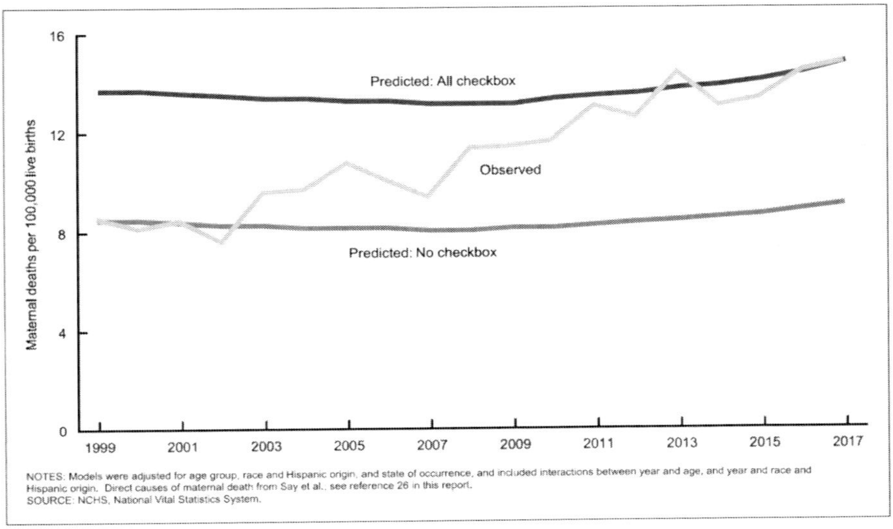

Figure A-I. Observed and predicted maternal mortality rates for direct causes of maternal death: United States, 1999–2017.

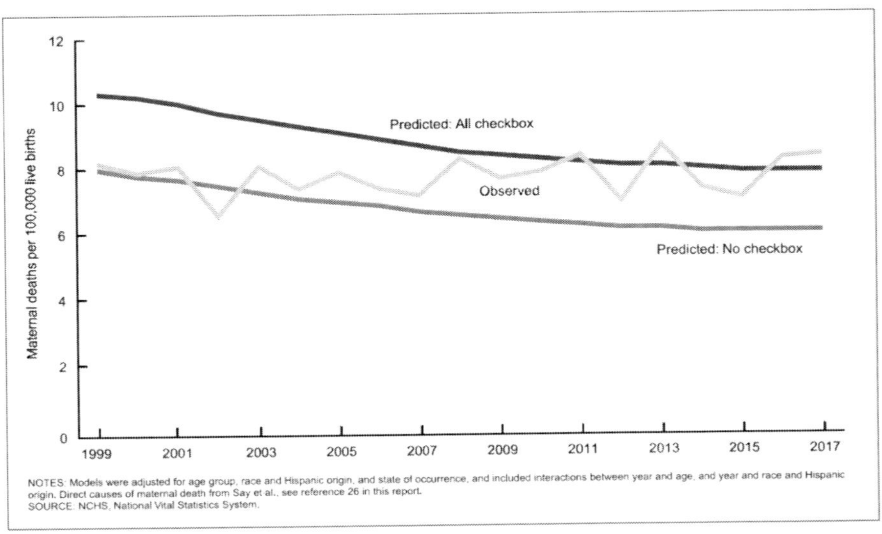

Figure A-II. Observed and predicted maternal mortality rates for direct causes of maternal death, excluding O26.8: United States, 1999–2017.

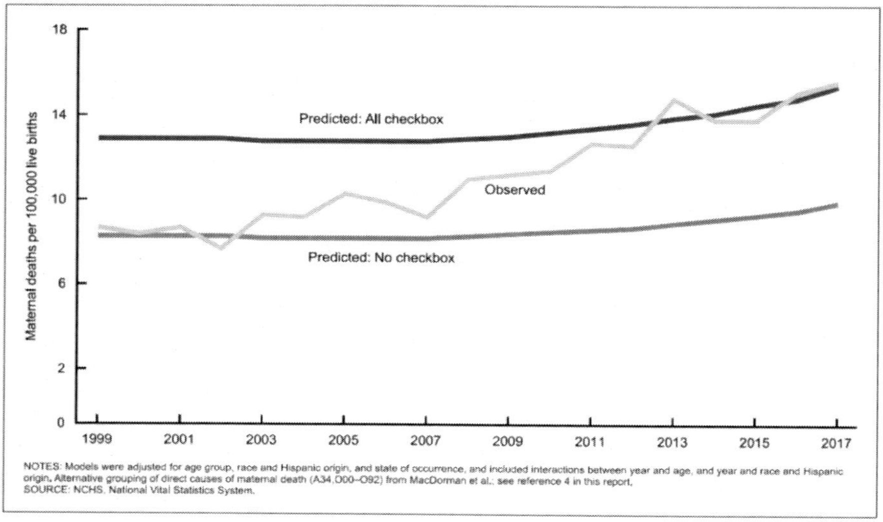

Figure A-III. Observed and predicted maternal mortality rates for direct causes of maternal death (A34, O00–O92): United States, 1999–2017.

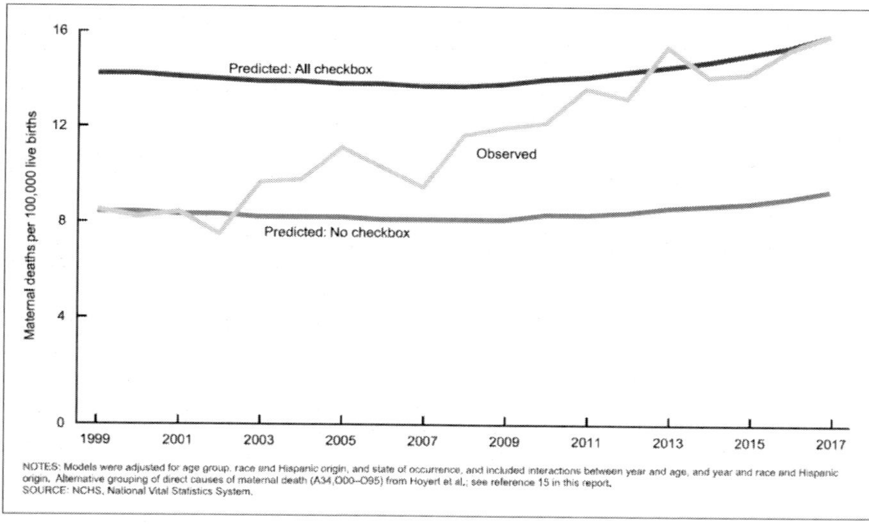

Figure A-IV. Observed and predicted maternal mortality rates for direct causes of maternal death (A34, O00–O95): United States, 1999–2017.

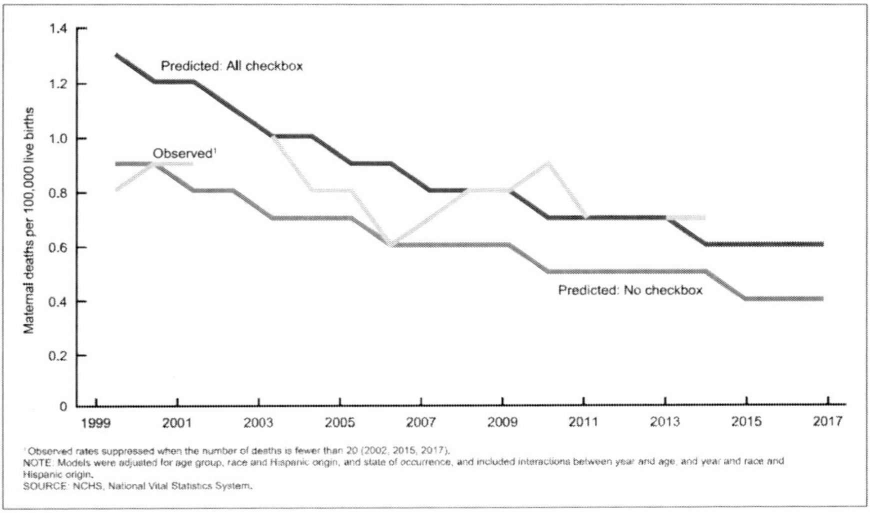

Figure A-V. Observed and predicted maternal mortality rates for pregnancy with abortive outcomes (O00–O07): United States, 1999–2017.

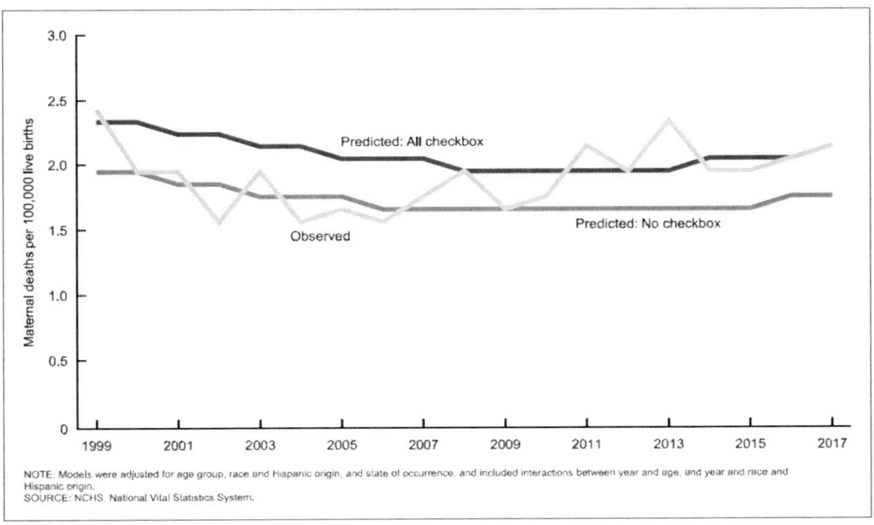

Figure A-VI. Observed and predicted maternal mortality rates for edema, proteinuria, and hypertensive disorders in pregnancy, childbirth, and the puerperium (O10–O16): United States, 1999–2017.

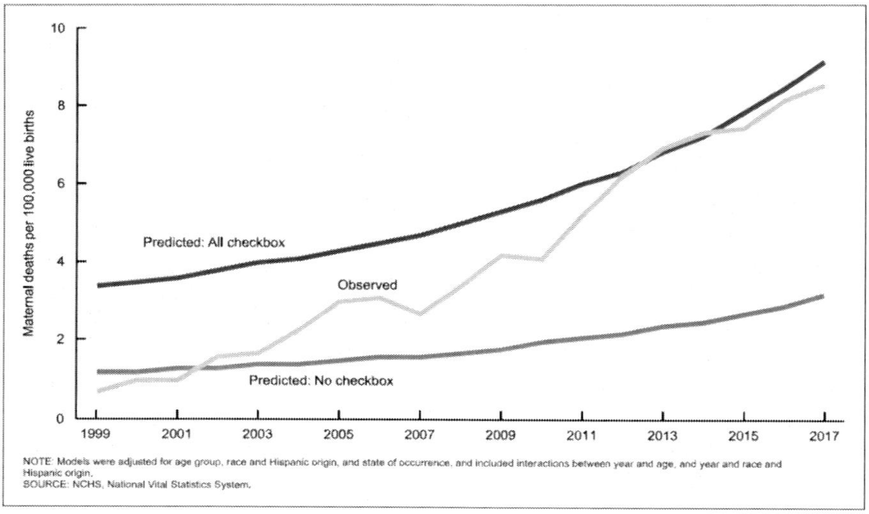

Figure A-VII. Observed and predicted maternal mortality rates for other maternal disorders predominantly related to pregnancy (O20–O29): United States, 1999–2017.

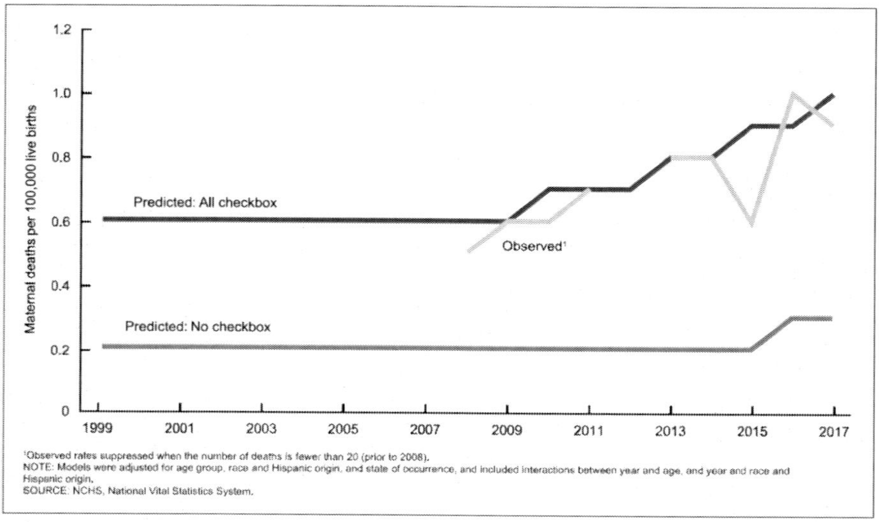

Figure A-VIII. Observed and predicted maternal mortality rates for liver disorders in pregnancy, childbirth, and the puerperium (O26.6): United States, 1999–2017.

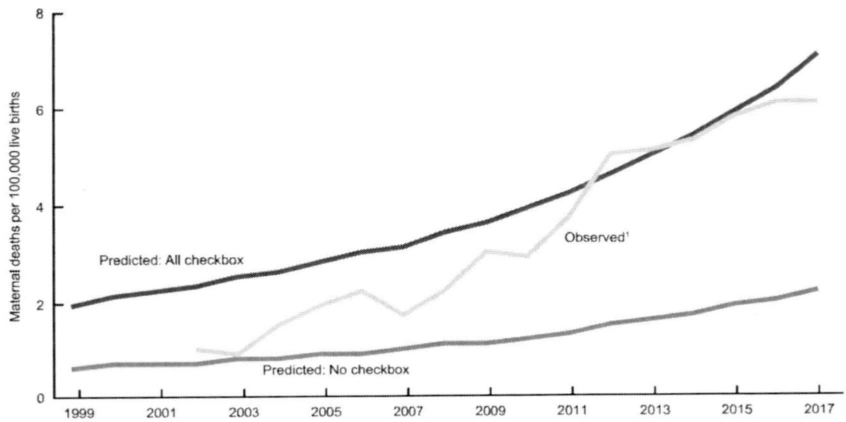

[1]Observed rates suppressed when the number of deaths is fewer than 20 (prior to 2002).
NOTE: Models were adjusted for age group, race and Hispanic origin, and state of occurrence, and included interactions between year and age, and year and race and Hispanic origin.
SOURCE: NCHS, National Vital Statistics System.

Figure A-IX. Observed and predicted maternal mortality rates for other specified pregnancy-related conditions (O26.8): United States, 1999–2017.

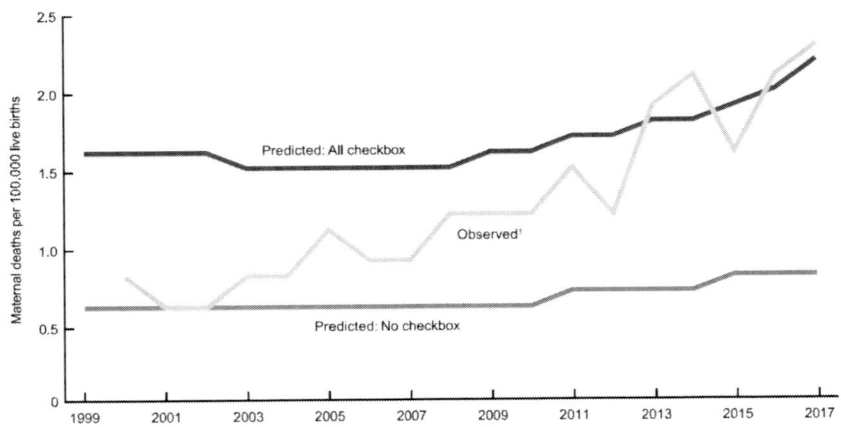

[1]Observed rates suppressed when the number of deaths is fewer than 20 (1999).
NOTE: Models were adjusted for age group, race and Hispanic origin, and state of occurrence, and included interactions between year and age, and year and race and Hispanic origin.
SOURCE: NCHS, National Vital Statistics System.

Figure A-X. Observed and predicted maternal mortality rates for other maternal disorders predominantly related to pregnancy (O20–O29), excluding nonspecific O26.8: United States, 1999–2017.

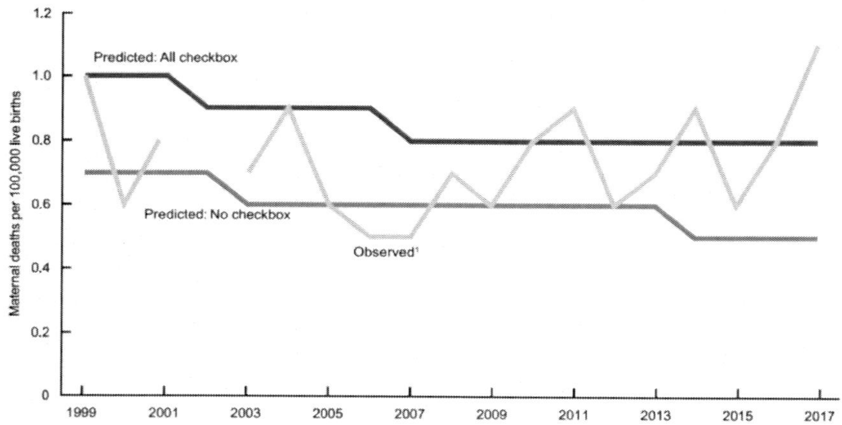

[1]Observed rates suppressed when the number of deaths is fewer than 20 (2002).
NOTE: Models were adjusted for age group, race and Hispanic origin, and state of occurrence, and included interactions between year and age, and year and race and Hispanic origin.
SOURCE: NCHS, National Vital Statistics System.

Figure A-XI. Observed and predicted maternal mortality rates for maternal care related to the fetus and amniotic cavity and possible delivery problems (O30–O48): United States, 1999–2017.

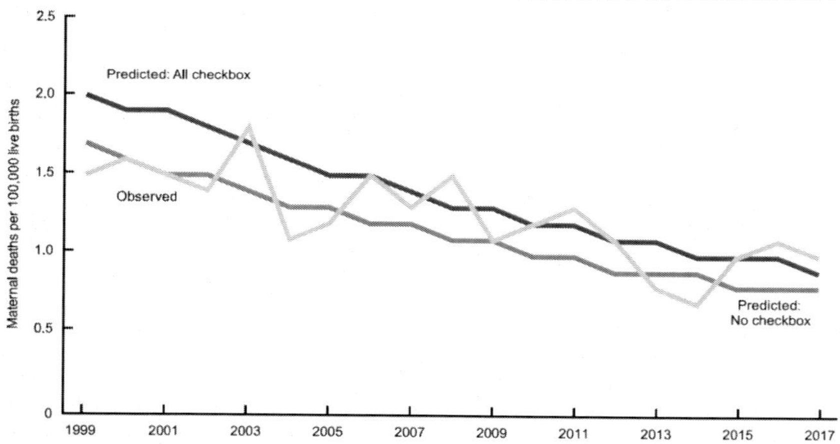

NOTE: Models were adjusted for age group, race and Hispanic origin, and state of occurrence, and included interactions between year and age, and year and race and Hispanic origin.
SOURCE: NCHS, National Vital Statistics System

Figure A-XII. Observed and predicted maternal mortality rates for complications of labor and delivery (O60–O75): United States, 1999–2017.

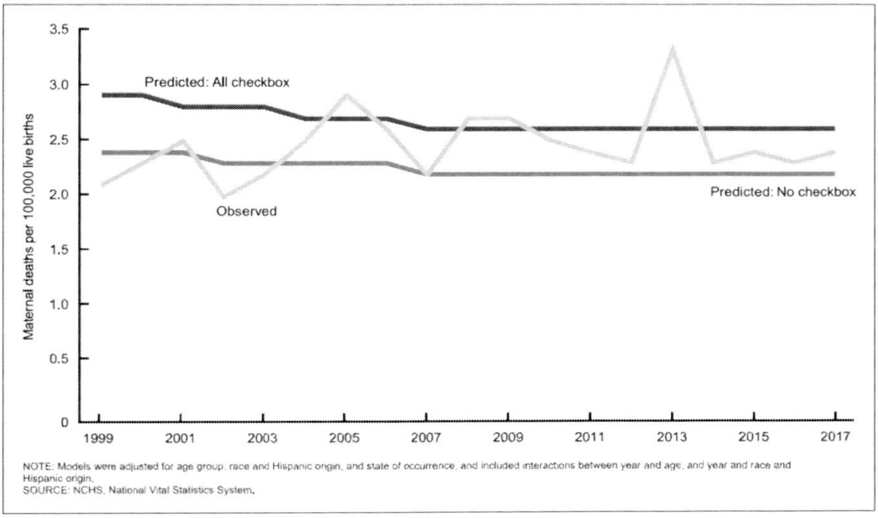

Figure A-XIII. Observed and predicted maternal mortality rates for complications predominantly related to the puerperium (O85–O92): United States, 1999–2017.

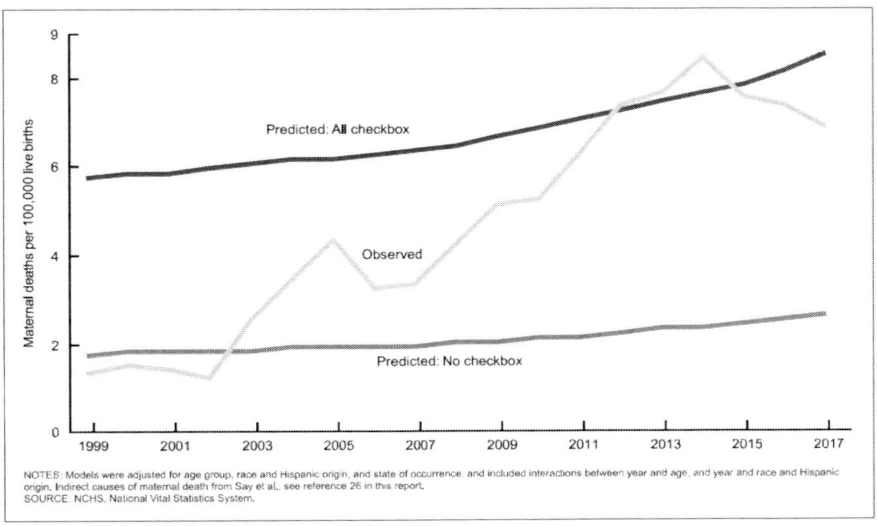

Figure A-XIV. Observed and predicted maternal mortality rates for indirect causes of maternal death: United States, 1999–2017.

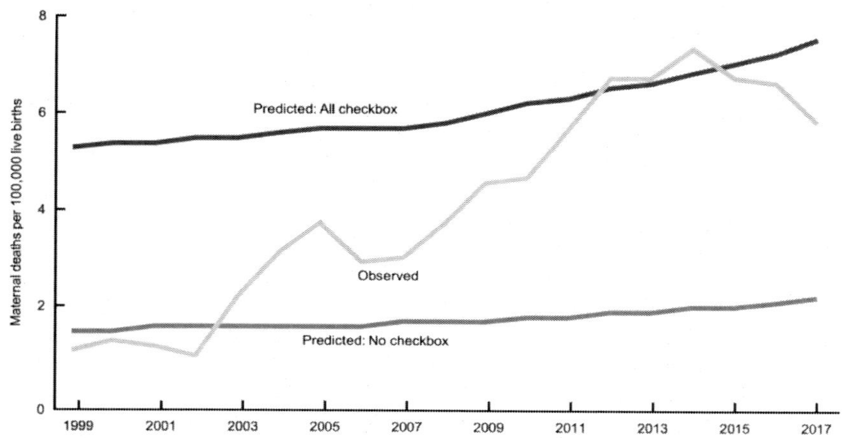

NOTES: Models were adjusted for age group, race and Hispanic origin, and state of occurrence, and included interactions between year and age, and year and race and Hispanic origin. Alternative grouping of indirect causes of maternal death (O98–O99) from MacDorman et al.; see reference 4 in this report.
SOURCE: NCHS, National Vital Statistics System.

Figure A-XV. Observed and predicted maternal mortality rates for alternative grouping of indirect causes of maternal death (O98–O99): United States, 1999–2017.

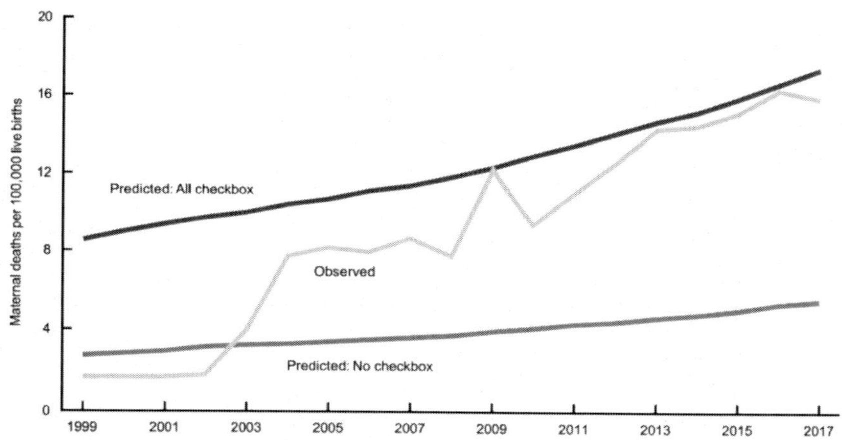

NOTE: Models were adjusted for age group, race and Hispanic origin, and state of occurrence, and included interactions between year and age, and year and race and Hispanic origin.
SOURCE: NCHS, National Vital Statistics System.

Figure A-XVI. Observed and predicted maternal mortality rates for other obstetric conditions not elsewhere classified, including late maternal deaths (O95–O99): United States, 1999–2017.

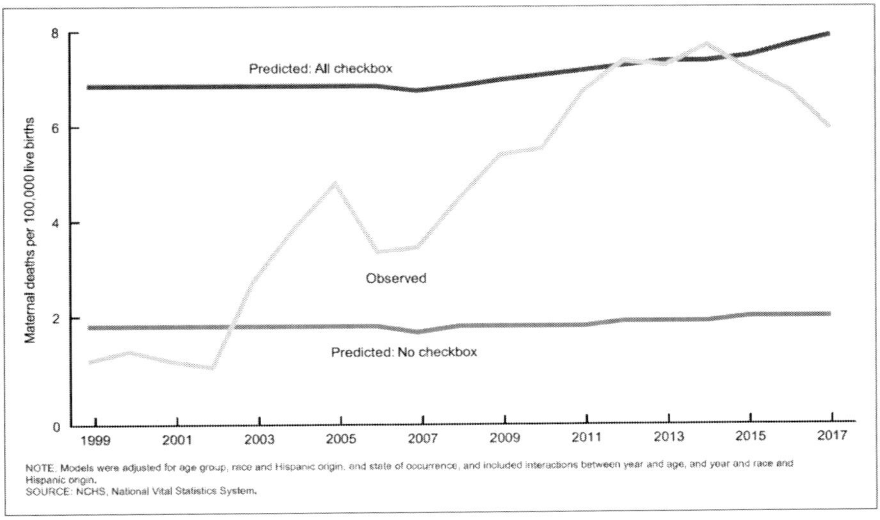

Figure A-XVII. Observed and predicted maternal mortality rates for other obstetric conditions not elsewhere classified, excluding late maternal deaths (O95, O98–O99): United States, 1999–2017.

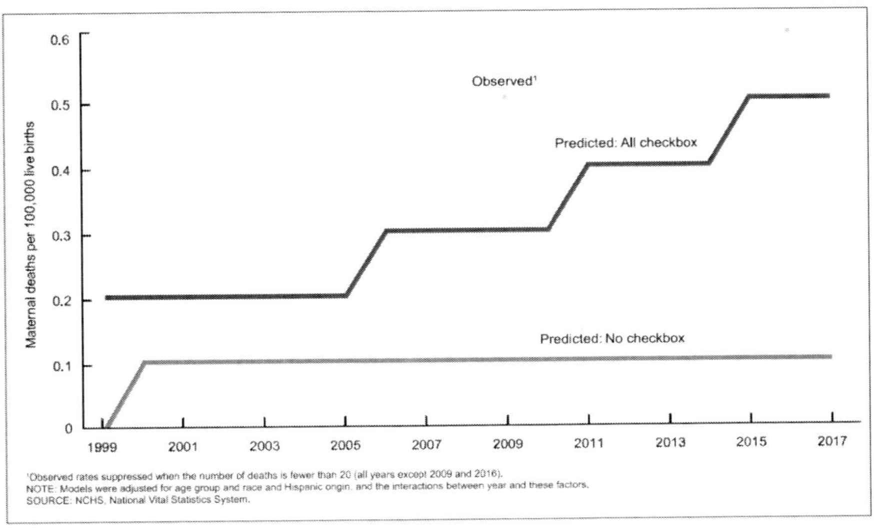

Figure A-XVIII. Observed and predicted maternal mortality rates for mental disorders and diseases of the nervous system complicating pregnancy, childbirth, and the puerperium (O99.3): United States, 1999–2017.

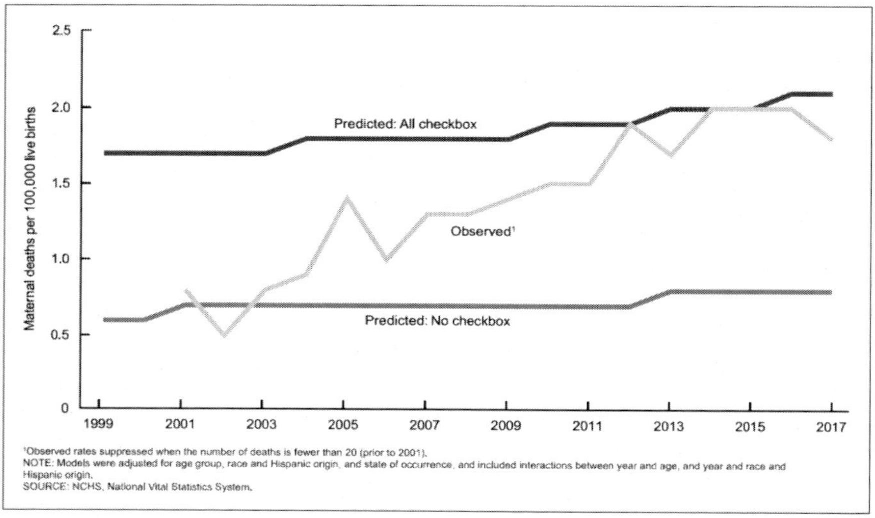

Figure A-XIX. Observed and predicted maternal mortality rates for diseases of the circulatory system complicating pregnancy, childbirth, and the puerperium (O99.4): United States, 1999–2017.

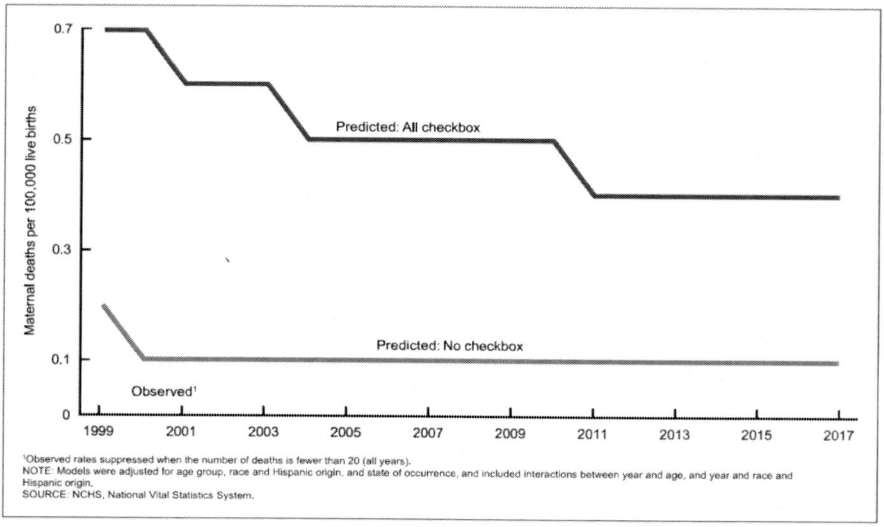

Figure A-XX. Observed and predicted maternal mortality rates for diseases of the respiratory system complicating pregnancy, childbirth, and the puerperium (O99.5): United States, 1999–2017.

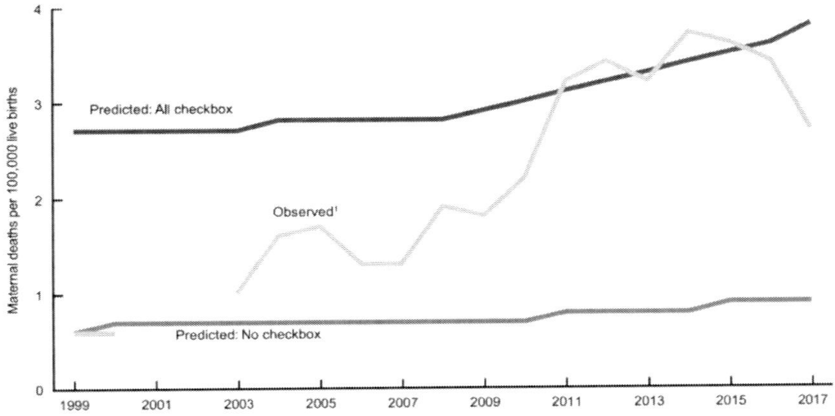

[1]Observed rates suppressed when the number of deaths is fewer than 20 (2001–2002).
NOTE: Models were adjusted for age group, race and Hispanic origin, and state of occurrence, and included interactions between year and age, and year and race and Hispanic origin.
SOURCE: NCHS, National Vital Statistics System.

Figure A-XXI. Observed and predicted maternal mortality rates for other specified diseases and conditions complicating pregnancy, childbirth, and the puerperium (O99.8): United States, 1999–2017.

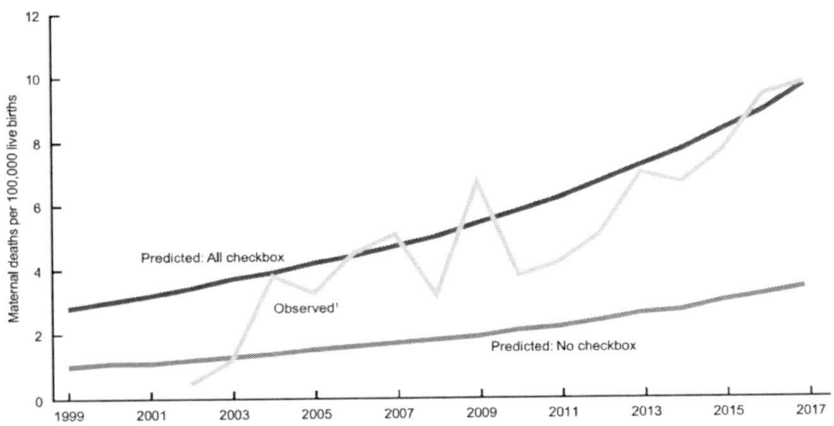

[1]Observed rates suppressed when the number of deaths is fewer than 20 (prior to 2002).
NOTE: Models were adjusted for age group, race and Hispanic origin, and state of occurrence, and included interactions between year and age, and year and race and Hispanic origin.
SOURCE: NCHS, National Vital Statistics System.

Figure A-XXII. Observed and predicted maternal mortality rates for late maternal deaths (O96–O97): United States, 1999–2017.

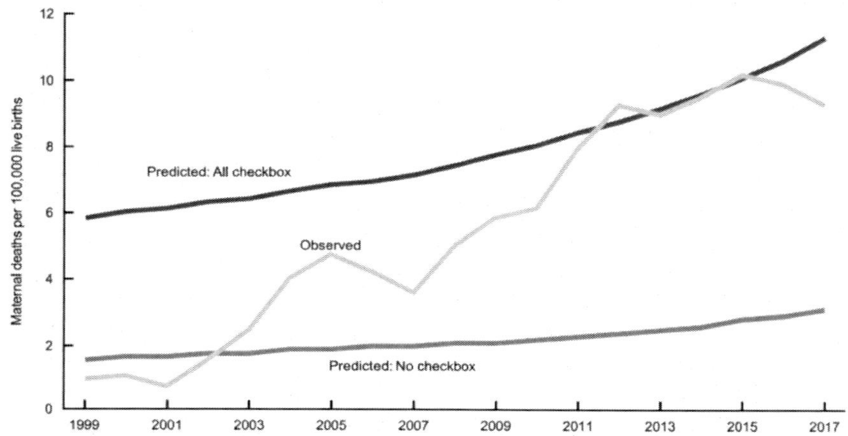

NOTE: Models were adjusted for age group, race and Hispanic origin, and state of occurrence, and included interactions between year and age, and year and race and Hispanic origin.
SOURCE: NCHS, National Vital Statistics System.

Figure A-XXIII. Observed and predicted maternal mortality rates for nonspecific causes of maternal death (O26.8, O95, O99.8): United States, 1999–2017.

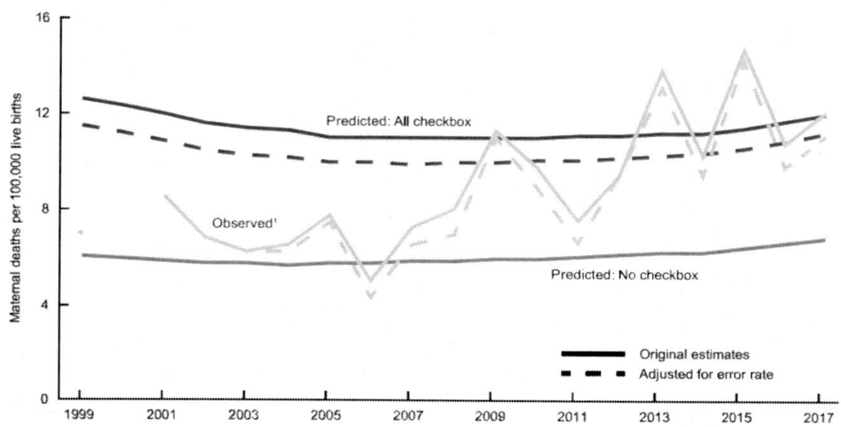

[1]Observed rates suppressed when the number of deaths is fewer than 20 (2000).
NOTES: Dotted lines represent maternal mortality rates (MMRs) adjusted for fixed error rates, while solid lines depict the original predicted and observed MMRs. Models were adjusted for age group, race and Hispanic origin, and state of occurrence, and included interactions between these factors and year as well as revision status.
SOURCE: NCHS, National Vital Statistics System.

Figure A-XXIV. Observed and predicted maternal mortality rates among females aged 15–19, adjusted for an error rate of 0.50% in the pregnancy checkbox: United States, 1999–2017.

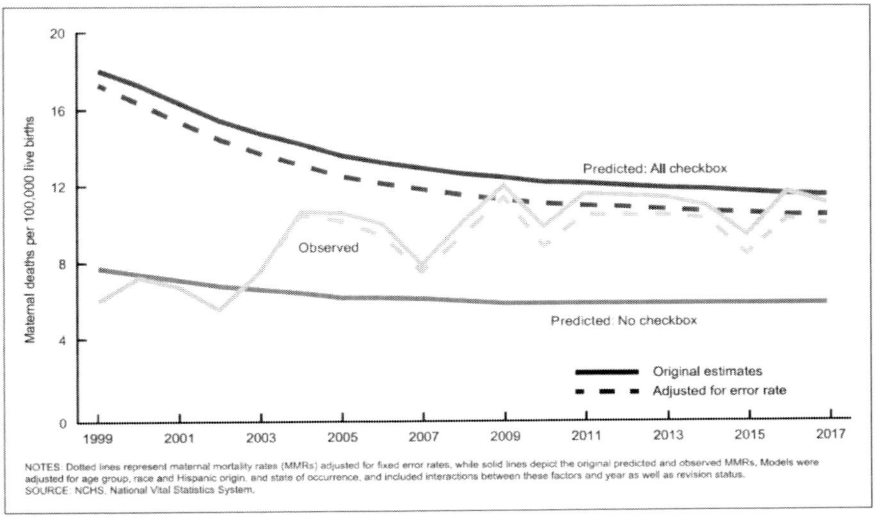

Figure A-XXV. Observed and predicted maternal mortality rates among women aged 20–24, adjusted for an error rate of 0.50% in the pregnancy checkbox: United States, 1999–2017.

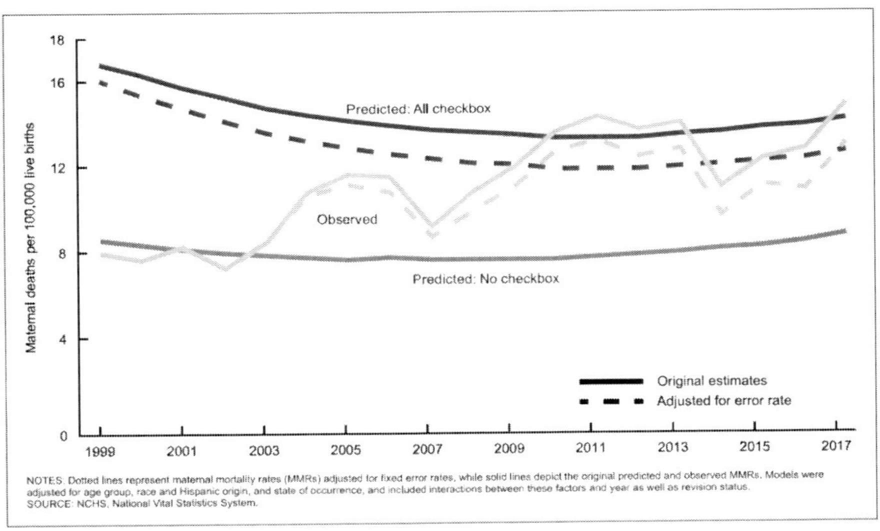

Figure A-XXVI. Observed and predicted maternal mortality rates among women aged 25–29, adjusted for an error rate of 0.50% in the pregnancy checkbox: United States, 1999–2017.

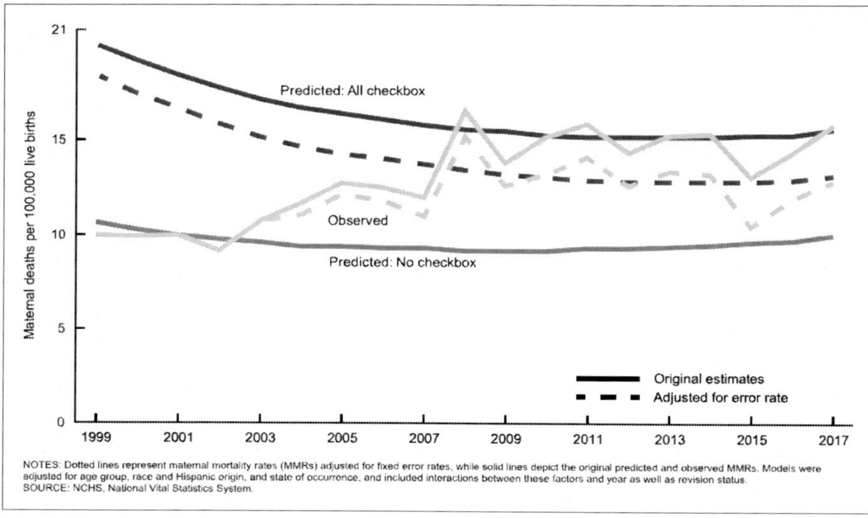

Figure A-XXVII. Observed and predicted maternal mortality rates among women aged 30–34, adjusted for an error rate of 0.50% in the pregnancy checkbox: United States, 1999–2017.

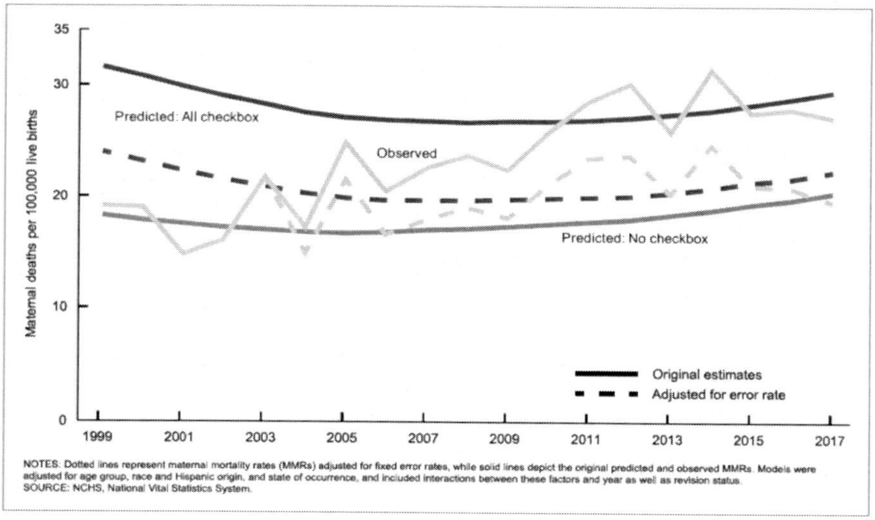

Figure A-XXVIII. Observed and predicted maternal mortality rates among women aged 35–39, adjusted for an error rate of 0.50% in the pregnancy checkbox: United States, 1999–2017.

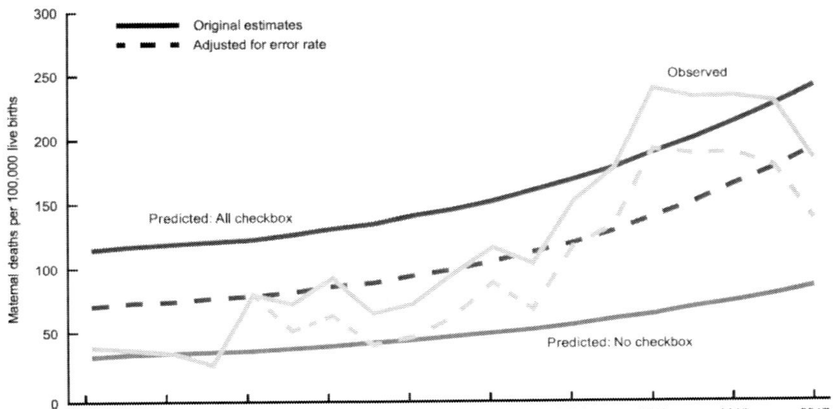

NOTES: Dotted lines represent maternal mortality rates (MMRs) adjusted for fixed error rates, while solid lines depict the original predicted and observed MMRs. Models were adjusted for age group, race and Hispanic origin, and state of occurrence, and included interactions between these factors and year as well as revision status.
SOURCE: NCHS, National Vital Statistics System.

Figure A-XXIX. Observed and predicted maternal mortality rates among women aged 40 and over, adjusted for an error rate of 0.50% in the pregnancy checkbox: United States, 1999–2017.

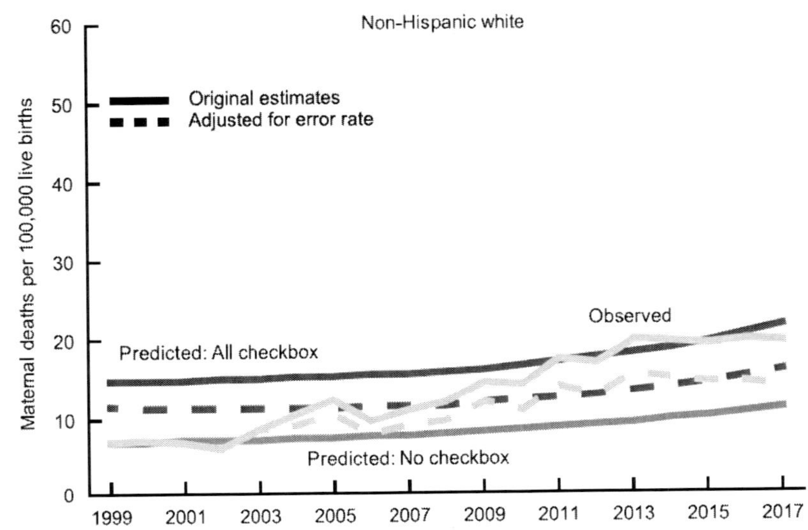

Figure A-XXX. (Continued).

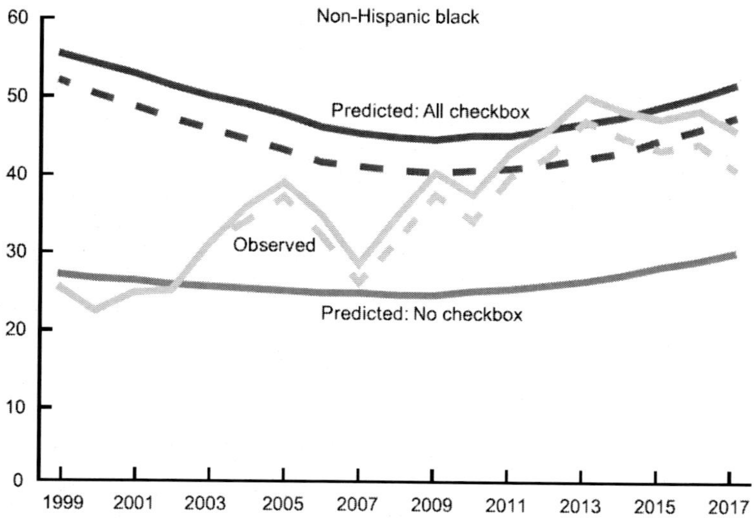

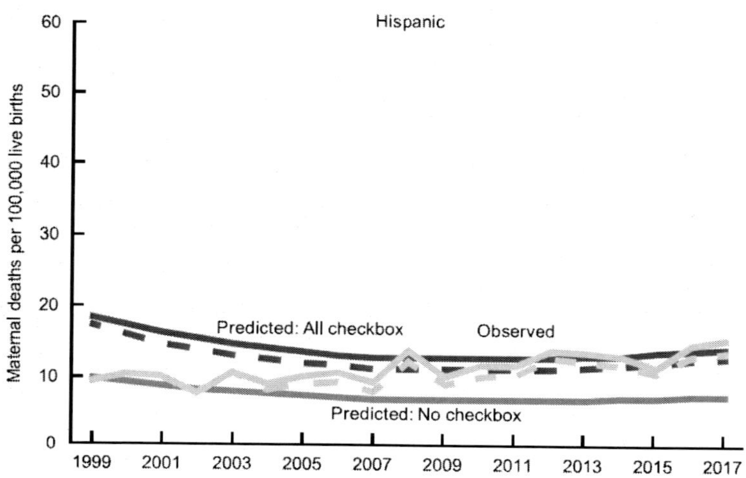

Figure A-XXX. (Continued).

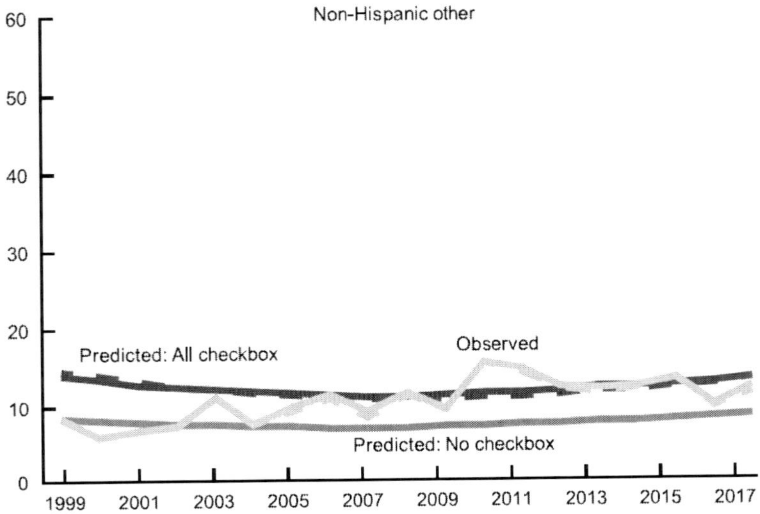

Note: Models were adjusted for age group, race and Hispanic origin, and state of occurrence, and included interactions between these factors and year as well as revision status.

Source: NCHS, National Vital Statistics System.

Figure A-XXX. Observed and predicted maternal mortality rates, by race and Hispanic origin, adjusted for an error rate of 0.50% in the pregnancy checkbox: United States, 1999–2017.

VITAL AND HEALTH STATISTICS SERIES DESCRIPTIONS

Active Series

Series 1. Programs and Collection Procedures

Reports describe the programs and data systems of the National Center for Health Statistics, and the data collection and survey methods used. Series 1 reports also include definitions, survey design, estimation, and other material necessary for understanding and analyzing the data.

Series 2. Data Evaluation and Methods Research

Reports present new statistical methodology including experimental tests of new survey methods, studies of vital and health statistics collection methods, new analytical techniques, objective evaluations of reliability of collected data, and contributions to statistical theory. Reports also include comparison of U.S. methodology with those of other countries.

Series 3. Analytical and Epidemiological Studies

Reports present data analyses, epidemiological studies, and descriptive statistics based on national surveys and data systems. As of 2015, Series 3 includes reports that would have previously been published in Series 5, 10–15, and 20–23.

Discontinued Series

Series 4. Documents and Committee Reports

Reports contain findings of major committees concerned with vital and health statistics and documents. The last Series 4 report was published in 2002; these are now included in Series 2 or another appropriate series.

Series 5. International Vital and Health Statistics Reports

Reports present analytical and descriptive comparisons of U.S. vital and health statistics with those of other countries. The last Series 5 report was published in 2003; these are now included in Series 3 or another appropriate series.

Series 6. Cognition and Survey Measurement

Reports use methods of cognitive science to design, evaluate, and test survey instruments. The last Series 6 report was published in 1999; these are now included in Series 2.

Series 10. Data from the National Health Interview Survey

Reports present statistics on illness; accidental injuries; disability; use of hospital, medical, dental, and other services; and other health-related topics. As of 2015, these are included in Series 3.

Series 11. Data from the National Health Examination Survey, the National Health and Nutrition Examination Surveys, and the Hispanic Health and Nutrition Examination Survey

Reports present 1) estimates of the medically defined prevalence of specific diseases in the United States and the distribution of the population with respect to physical, physiological, and psychological characteristics and 2) analysis of relationships among the various measurements. As of 2015, these are included in Series 3.

Series 12. Data from the Institutionalized Population Surveys

The last Series 12 report was published in 1974; these reports were included in Series 13, and as of 2015 are in Series 3.

Series 13. Data from the National Health Care Survey

Reports present statistics on health resources and use of health care resources based on data collected from health care providers and provider records. As of 2015, these reports are included in Series 3.

Series 14. Data on Health Resources: Manpower and Facilities

The last Series 14 report was published in 1989; these reports were included in Series 13, and are now included in Series 3.

Series 15. Data from Special Surveys

Reports contain statistics on health and health-related topics from surveys that are not a part of the continuing data systems of the National Center for Health Statistics. The last Series 15 report was published in 2002; these reports are now included in Series 3.

Series 16. Compilations of Advance Data from Vital and Health Statistics

The last Series 16 report was published in 1996. All reports are available online; compilations are no longer needed.

Series 20. Data on Mortality

Reports include analyses by cause of death and demographic variables, and geographic and trend analyses. The last Series report was published in 2007; these reports are now included in Series 3.

Series 21. Data on Natality, Marriage, and Divorce

Reports include analyses by health and demographic variables, and geographic and trend analyses. The last Series report was published in 2006; these reports are now included in Series 3.

Series 22. Data from the National Mortality and Natality Surveys

The last Series 22 report was published in 1973. Reports from sample surveys of vital records were included in Series 20 or 21, and are now included in Series 3.

Series 23. Data from the National Survey of Family Growth

Reports contain statistics on factors that affect birth rates, factors affecting the formation and dissolution of families, and behavior related to the risk of HIV and other sexually transmitted diseases. The last Series 23 report was published in 2011; these reports are now included in Series 3.

Series 24. Compilations of Data on Natality, Mortality, Marriage, and Divorce

The last Series 24 report was published in 1996. All reports are available online; compilations are no longer needed.

INDEX

C

D

E

F

G

H

I

L

M

N

O

P

Q

R

S

T

U

W

Y